May this book be a true
blessing and inspiration

Cheers,
   the Randolphs

PURE 5:2
Transformation in 21 Days

Robyn & Geoff Randolph
2nd Edition

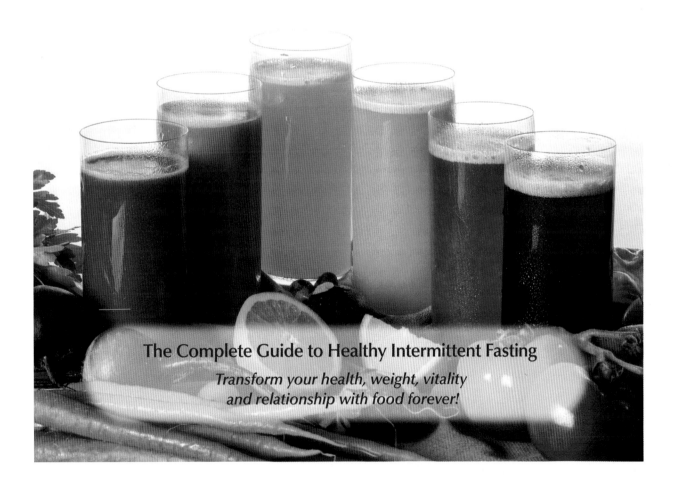

The Complete Guide to Healthy Intermittent Fasting

Transform your health, weight, vitality
and relationship with food forever!

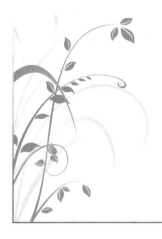

Dedication

This book is dedicated to the One who is our true compass in life and the source of our intuition, inspiration, and creativity.

Famous Food Quotes to Ponder

"To eat is a necessity, but to eat intelligently is an art."
— *La Rochefoucauld*

"Those who think they have no time for healthy eating will sooner or later have to find time for illness."
— *Edward Stanley (1826–1893) from The Conduct of Life*

"When you fast... your Father shall reward you openly."
— *Matthew 6:17–18*

"Daniel made up his mind he would not defile himself with the king's meat and wine... Let us be given pulses to eat, and water to drink... At the end of ten days, their appearance was handsomer, and they were stronger, than all the youths who had been eating the king's food."
— *Daniel 1:12–20*

"The doctor of the future will give no medicine, but will interest his patients in the care of human frame, and in the cause and prevention of disease."
— *T. A. Edison*

"Today, more than 95% of all chronic disease is caused by food choice, toxic food ingredients, nutritional deficiencies and lack of physical exercise."
— *Mike Adams, author, investigative journalist, and educator*

"Tell me what you eat, and I will tell you who you are."
— *Brillat-Savarin*

"One should eat to live, not live to eat."
— *Benjamin Franklin*

"We never repent of having eaten too little."
— *Thomas Jefferson*

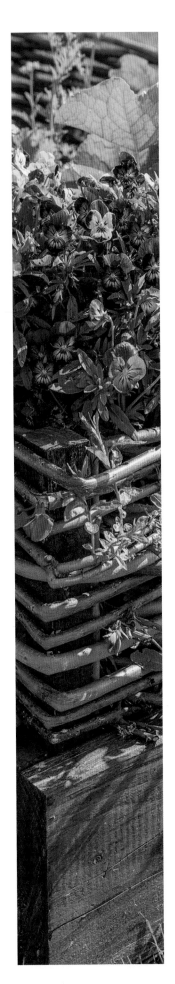

Important Disclaimer and Warning:

The information in this book is intended to be informative and in no way used as a diagnosis or prescription. When changing your diet or exercise regime, we suggest that you seek appropriate wise counsel from your doctor or health care professional, first.

The author, publisher and distributors of this book are not responsible for any changes in your body as a result of your choice to implement anything suggested in writing within the pages of this book.

The intention of this information and these recipes is to inspire you to make healthy choices, to encourage you to enjoy the art and delight of healthful food preparation and to educate you about the tremendous benefits of eating pure and raw, whole foods.

WARNING: Fasting is strictly off limits for those who are pregnant, diabetic, anyone who suffers from kidney or liver disease or persons on prescription drugs. Intermittent fasting is very popular right now. Sadly we see many people attempting this, thinking they can eat whatever they want (processed, GMO, irradiated, packaged, fast foods) on the 5 days and then jump into fasting days with coffee, water and/or high sugar content juices. If you think you can eat toxic food 5 days a week and fast for 2 days a week and not face toxic withdrawal results and negative body reactions, think again. If you have hypoglycemia, this book will help you in many ways to understand your next steps. We suggest you learn about eating PURE and work on getting balanced and healed before going for long stretches of time without eating. Read on to find out how to get the healthiest results for your unique body and circumstances.

A special thank you to Iris Richardson, irisrichardson.com; Su Gatch, sugraphics.com; and Lynda Benham, Marianne Wyllie and Eric Randoph for their editing and proofing. A special thank you to Stuart of Tyson Press for bending over backwards with publishing this edition in hard copy. What an amazing, talented team and joy to work with. Thank you to David Sandoval, author of *The Green Food Bible* and CEO of our favorite source for the purest, premium food supplements, Purium Health Products! Your wisdom and inspiration is timeless and has made such a difference in our lives! We also want to thank Dr. Mercola for doing such a tremendous job educating the world about healthy eating and living. We appreciate your perspectives and value your continued dedication to reporting about the latest cutting edge information.

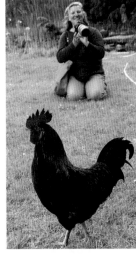

Published and distributed by:

Pure Highland Living

All photography by Iris Richardson unless otherwise noted.

Table of Contents

Table of Contents, continued

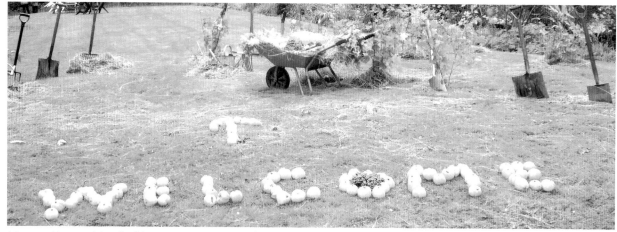

Harvest Fete at Newbold House, Forres, Scotland

Introduction

PURE Food Revival

Wake up and smell the fresh juice. Wakie, wakie…no more eggs and bac-ie! (As in, processed nitrate bacon).

This book is about finding and eating PURE food in a toxic world. No matter if you are a carnivore, vegetarian or vegan, perhaps following the Paleo Diet, Raw Food Cuisine, Intermittent Fasting and/or Intuitive Eating as lifestyle choices, the pressing issue at hand for everyone is finding food that truly nourishes us in a form that is easy to acquire and prepare. People today have access to food and "food-like substances" like never before, yet they are starving for true nutrition.

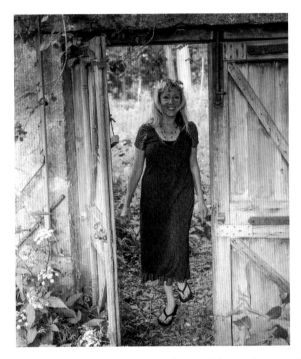

In this book you will find a wealth of information (and delicious, nutrient-dense recipes) whether you decide to do Intermittent Fasting or not.

We have investigated and reported on the overwhelming fact that diseases and obesity are skyrocketing for young and old, far and wide, in historical proportions. We are facing the consequences of big business, marketing and a system that has led us over the cliff of health and well-being.

Clearly there is something bigger than our passion on this topic driving us to write this book. Each page and chapter was crafted from a voice that represents our (all those drawn to read this book) collective cries for help.

When I was poisoned, seventeen years ago, I remember that incapacitated state of toxic overload searing my every fiber. I still have not forgotten for a minute what it was like to feel so helpless, so worn down. Amidst the overwhelm and foggy brain, I had to learn how to eat PURE to recover.

While writing this book, a close family member was diagnosed with cancer. My heart deeply empathizes now as she is scrambling to make up for lost time and relearn how to nourish herself well so she can eat PURE to live well.

As we wrote, each chapter emerged from a momentum and heartbeat of a collective awareness that is pulsing for revival. A revival of what was once known, and a way of sustainable nourishment that made up the underpinnings of life as the seasons carried people across the planes of existence.

The word *revival* means an instance of something becoming popular, active, or important again.

The answers to our health, obesity and blood sugar issues do not come from those who have poisoned us. The answers come from what created us. We need to learn from the past to walk more fully into our future. In slowing down and listening, we have a lot to learn from our own intuition as well as from our ancestors, who walked this world before us in health and in metabolically balanced, trim bodies…

Those Paleo-people knew how to live, eat, and thrive season after season, eating organic, locally and sustainably!

We have merged both Intermittent Fasting and Intuitive Eating because we feel that these concepts give people practical ways to transform their understanding and relationship with food.

Moreover, this is the way our bodies have been designed to operate over countless eons. It is abnormal to live in a state of constant food surplus wed with sedentary lifestyles. Our bodies are designed to handle fluctuations in food availability and intake; they require that to remain healthy.

Intermittent Fasting is a very popular concept in today's weight loss trends. However, we find the benefits of eating a PURE 5:2 diet far exceeds weight loss. Adopting the suggestions we have outlined in this book will take you to a wholesome new level of health and wellness. When applied properly, this book provides the tools to support you to detox, cleanse, and regenerate. We have also included information on cancer and radiation prevention. In a time when radiation fallout from Fukushima is a global wake-up call, it is necessary for us all to be educated about the health risks we face as well as the dietary precautions we can take.

We offer you this book as a tool for understanding and for transformation. If this makes sense to you and intuitively resonates as truth, then we encourage you to take 21 Days to put into practice PURE 5:2 Transformation using the information and step-by-step guidance in these pages.

Although we may feel powerless and overwhelmed in a toxic world filled with chemicals, lobbyists and big businesses enabled by deceitful politicians…we can empower ourselves every day and every meal with the choices we make and the foods we buy. This is how we can make a difference, personally and collectively. The time is now for a PURE Food Revival.©

We sincerely hope this book reaches every ear that will hear and heart that will share the truth about what is really going on with our food and how that is affecting all of us. We are grateful you are hungry for transformation and a PURE food revival.

With much gratitude,
Robyn and Geoff Randolph

To see what we are up to here in the highlands of Scotland see our You Tube video: **Real People, Pure Food…Revival Project** (on our Pure Highland Living Channel).

For speaking engagements, personal or group retreats, or healthy holiday workshops, email us at: **purehighlandliving@gmail.com**

To purchase more copies of this book please send an email to: **purehighlandliving@gmail.com**

Please specifiy if you would like an autographed copy and who you would like it made out to. Retail and wholesale prices available.

Visit our websites for free recipes, information and how to purchase supplies and equipment:

UK and USA:
purehighlandliving.com and
kaleconsciousness.com

USA only: **phporder.com/rawsome**

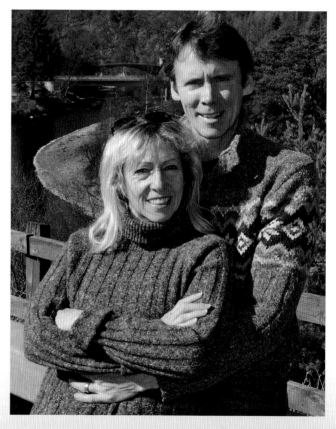

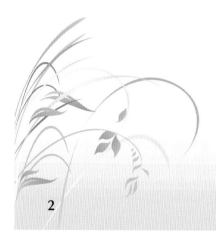

PART 1

CHAPTER 1 – Why PURE?

What to Expect from PURE 5:2 Transformation

Welcome to PURE 5:2! Whether you are a Paleo, raw foodist, vegan, vegetarian, pescetarian, or carnivore, this book is about inspiring and encouraging you to transform your relationship and results with food by learning how to use your intuition and intermittent fasting with RAW and SOME Cooked PURE foods (hence RawSome PURE Foods, also termed as PURE Revival Foods).

This book is about a transformative lifestyle, not about a diet. It is about learning how to really take care of yourself from the inside out, feeding yourself on an intuitive and cellular level, not deprivation or starvation. The focus is on optimal health, wellness, anti-aging, disease prevention and vitality, not on counting calories or dieting tricks to lose weight. People can learn to lose weight by doing simple math and yet still reap the havoc that comes from eating toxic foods. What good is it to shed pounds only to gain a weakened and diseased body?

In 21 days you can expect to:

- Find freedom from counting calories and dieting
- Enjoy finding satisfaction from eating less
- Stop food cravings and break the food addiction cycle
- Learn easy, nourishing recipes
- Feel greater energy and vitality
- Generally feel more balanced
- Get comfortable with new healthy habits that are sustainable
- Develop a new relationship with food that takes you to a wholesome new level
- Learn what foods in your diet can be upgraded to produce the results you are after

- Learn how and why to eat healthy PURE food as a lifestyle
- Focus on a healthy lifestyle, not weight management
- Feel less bloated
- Feel lighter
- Learn both traditional and raw food cooking methods for deeply nourishing results
- Feel healthier and more balanced energy
- Feel an overall enhancement in your mood and well-being
- Be delighted with your results
- Enjoy sharing your success with others

What Does P. U. R. E. Stand For?

PURE is an acronym that we use in two ways:

1. *Periodic Unrestricted and Restricted Eating*

Refers to a lifestyle whereby 5 days a week you eat a healthy balanced "intuitive diet" (meaning listening to cues and signals that tell you what is best for your own body... nourishing your body in ways that intuitively feel best and make the most sense in regards to optimal health for your unique body and circumstances). These "5 days" are unrestricted in that you are encouraged to eat healthy, PURE foods in the amounts and ways you intuitively feel is nourishing. We believe there is not just one diet for everyone. Some people do better with animal protein and others find vitality by being vegan. No matter what you choose, most everyone can benefit from adding a range of more raw foods in their diet.

On the other two days, foods are restricted. The focus on these days is about "intermittent fasting" using "PURE revival foods" that are extremely nutrient dense, cleansing, and nourishing; foods that support the fasting process and are loaded with phytochemicals and antioxidants.

NOTE: It all depends on what your focus and goals are. On "2 days" the focus does not have to be totally about fasting. Some people use "2 days" to learn to juice and/or eat all raw, vegan while "fasting" from cooked and animal foods.

2. *Phytonutrients Unprocessed Raw and Enzyme-rich*

Refers to the attributes of the food we are suggesting you focus on incorporating into your daily diet. These foods revive our health as well as take us back to eating the way we were designed to eat before man-made, processed foods were invented. We will discuss this further, in greater detail.

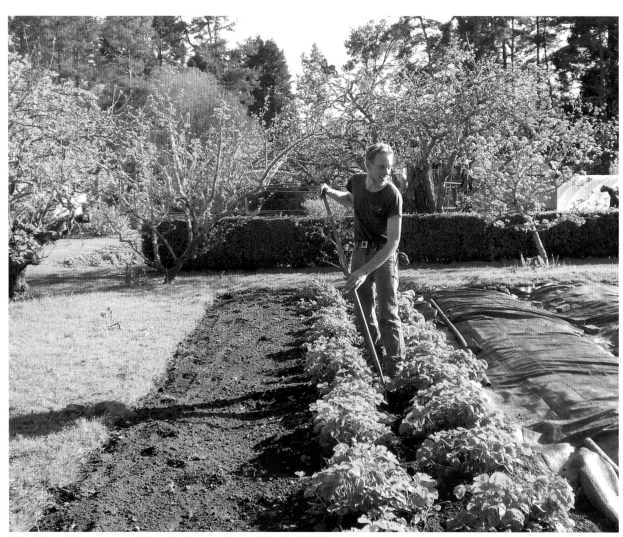

Our friend Lorenzo working in the garden at Newbold House

Our PURE Story

Robyn:

I grew up in Beverly Hills and let me tell you, that was no picnic. The picnic ended in fourth grade when I joined the ranks of girls over-focused on outward appearances. After all, wasn't that the real learning that was taking place, at my famous Beverly Hills High School, which later became the focus of a Hollywood TV show, "90210"?

In high school I tried dozens of fad diets. Who needed an amusement park when you could just ride the roller coaster of mood swings and fluctuating weight that binge eating and dieting produced! The goal was always to get skinny – no matter what it took.

I felt like a player on a board game. Go to lunch with friends. Eat all the carbs possible without "losing your cookies" (I didn't binge and purge). Drink diet cola to cut some corners. Undo the top button of your jeans and complain all afternoon about how fat you feel. Stir up enough drama to motivate yourself to go on a grapefruit diet the next day.

Starve yourself, except for half a grapefruit — eat a tiny triangular bit once an hour. At night, allow yourself to eat another grapefruit one section at a time, savoring every morsel. Do not pass Go, do not collect any money OR lose any weight... go straight to diet jail where you feel guilty for binging, yet again! Live off the fumes of binge, guilt, and remorse.

I grew up with a big daddy; I'm talking whopping big. He taught us to think about or eat food, almost all the time! If it wasn't mealtime, it was snack time or tea time or time for a cigarette break! He eventually ate his way to diabetes and colon cancer and died an obese man.

I was raised on a diet of fast foods, additives and preservatives. At age ten I was receiving Demerol injections to combat debilitating migraines. I was constantly sick with all kinds of immune issues. By the time I was eighteen, I was addicted to nasal spray and nicotine. I developed hypoglycemia, and at times would lose my vision and hearing, or pass out. Sometimes I ate as many as three times in the night just to make it through to morning. I have had Epstein Barr, glandular fever/mono, chronic fatigue, extreme candida and also suffered with severe anxiety attacks.

When I was forty, I was poisoned by off-gassing oil-based paint. I spent six hours on an IV in the hospital and was sent home with fistfuls of pills. People had to feed me, and at times I couldn't even open my eyes. For months, I barely made it through each day, each hour, each minute. When doctors had no solutions, I literally had to pray my way through each day.

> *I spent six hours on an IV in the hospital and was sent home with fistfuls of pills. At times, people had to feed me, and I couldn't even open my eyes.*

By amazing grace, highly focused research, trial and error, and hours of creative kitchen episodes, I found my way through the maze of intense body symptoms. Miraculously, I was led in the form of insights and impressions that came to me, one step at a time. Eating a balance of raw and cooked, and the specific PURE foods you will learn about in this book, laid the foundation for my recovery on a cellular level. People who were feeding me when I was so ill saw me slowly work my way through layers of toxicity and back to the land of the living.

Through juicing, carefully implementing specific high nutrient density foods and all-raw eating, I began to recover my strength and energy. Recipes filled my head and poured forth! I was inspired to put together all kinds of RawSome PURE recipes (some all-RAW and SOME cooked). Glorious energy and vitality seemed to be birthed from each new, inspired creation! Along with this came a new ability to be still and listen to my body.

Amidst my desperation, I sensed a deep, intuitive part of myself emerging. Cloaked in the veil of sheer survival instincts, my intuitive self began to have a sense about how, when, and what I should try to fuel my wellness. At first I would get a general sense about things. In time, as I practiced listening to and acting on the cues I received, the directives got more specific.

There was a point in my recovery where I was all-raw, vegan and puffed up about being so. Out of nowhere I received a strong, intuitive push: "Eat a hard boiled egg."

"Be gone, you non-vegan apparition from my past," I pleaded. However, the directive remained, and turned into an order: "You must eat a hard boiled egg."

Being very identified with my image as an all-raw person, I was convinced that if I ate an egg, I would slide down a slippery slope back into the perils of cooked foods — animal food at that! My recovery had come quite a ways at that point, yet I was at a plateau, unable to get past some tricky blood sugar issues.

As I listened to and followed my intuition about what and when I should eat, I also practiced harnessing this ability when creating recipes. I would intuitively sense the exact amounts of individual ingredients and from there, what foods would blend well with what. I had two criteria for foods to blend well together: they had to taste good together as well as work synergistically to create more vitality.

I began to sense that certain foods would build up my immune system and others would tear it down. Some foods gave me more energy, while others seemed to be difficult for my body to process. Foods that required more work for my body delayed my healing.

The more I listened, the more ingredients and recipes flowed in. Recipes became more refined, and I began to see how important it was to use high-density, nutritious foods, rich in raw phytochemicals with intact enzymes, to optimally nourish my body.

When people saw me full of vitality again, they wanted to know what I was doing. They asked for the recipes and then wanted lessons. I began the first edition of *RawSome Recipes* and teaching "hands on" workshops in 1996.

Like a car, if we use high-grade gas and change the oil, we will have a smoother, longer ride than if we fill the vehicle with the cheap stuff. In my quest for recovery and my passionate pursuit of wellness, I had stumbled upon a deep well of intuitive knowledge that healed a hidden aspect

Eating a balance of raw and cooked, and the specific PURE foods you will learn about in this book laid the foundation for my recovery on a cellular level.

of myself that was unbalanced my whole life — my relationship with food. I didn't have a healthy relationship with food. I had lost respect for food and used it to mask my pain and feelings of powerlessness. I wanted food to replace my boredom and fill the gaps in my desire to love and be loved. I was in a vicious cycle of being addicted to it and controlled by it. I was out of balance, not just physically — I was acting out emotionally in my relationship with food. It took getting poisoned and being laid so low for me to begin to understand.

From those experiences, and seventeen years of teaching workshops and working one-on-one with people, I have developed Intuitive Eating Tools to support you in being free from dieting, food entrapment, and concerns over weight. In this book you will find coaching and instructions you can use for a successful PURE 5:2 Transformation in 21 days! By developing our own intuitive food sense, we can learn to tell what foods act as catalysts to enhance our immune system and state of health. Bottom line, PURE foods are essential for health and vitality.

I met Geoff (on **match.com**, believe it or not) in the summer of 2011. Both in our fifties and divorced after marriages spanning over twenty years, it was amazing to meet at this stage of life and share our mutual delight for all things related to living a healthy PURE lifestyle! Little did we know when we met that we would get married and move from California to live our dreams in the magical Highlands of Scotland in just over a year! Sounds like a match.com commercial!

Geoff:

I grew up in California and have been interested in healthy eating most of my life. As a child I was overweight, as a result of eating the standard American processed food diet of the 60s. Strict weight targets for high school wrestling led me to my passion for understanding how what we eat affects the way we look, feel and exist in our bodies. Recently, I lived for ten years on a ranch in the remote mountains of Northern California, where I learned to be self-sufficient. I grew a large amount of my fruits and vegetables, as well as raised chickens, goats, hogs, rabbits and sheep.

We have moved to Scotland to pursue our passion for living a sustainable life, being with and around people who share our delight in growing, harvesting and preparing organic food in all its glory, in a place where the air is clean and daily living is polite and sweetly satisfying.

The real issue for all of us is about finding PURE food, safe and able to deliver high nutrient density. This book is the blend of both of our voices, relaying years of our collective experiences and observations with the understanding of:

What, when, and how we eat affects who and what we are.

We hope this information inspires and blesses you in your journey to live a vibrant, healthy life… one PURE bite at a time! Give yourself the gift of experiencing the 21-day PURE Transformation following our guidelines and Intuitive Eating Coaching. We would love to hear from you about all the wonderful transformations taking place. We love sharing ideas and input on our website so feel free to submit your ideas, recipes, review of our book (on Amazon) etc.

Contact us at: **purehighlandliving@gmail.com**

Eat well and be well!
Cheers!

Robyn and Geoff Randolph

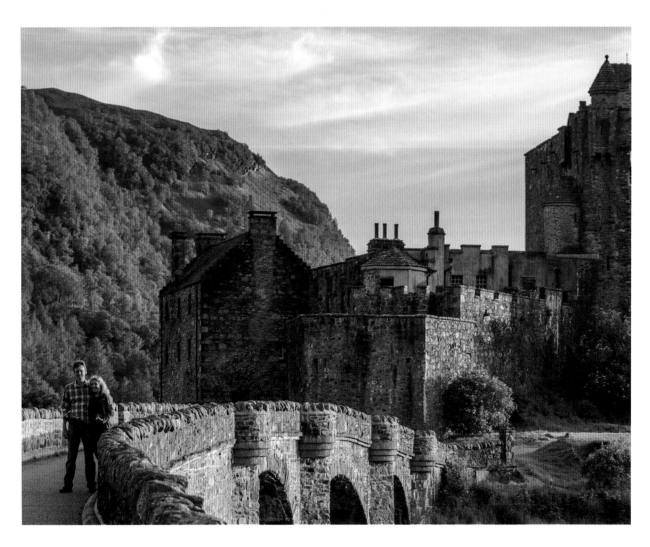

Where Did All the PURE Food Go?

"What is the perfect diet for me?" you might ask. "But I thought eating soy was good for me and what about that rapeseed/canola oil? Are protein powders really not good? What about the drawer full of expensive vitamins and supplements? Which foods are really providing 'superior' nutrition? All my favorite foods—they tell me are no good and now I can't even drink the water!!! Help!"

If you have ever dabbled even a little bit into the vast array of information out there about nutrition, you will agree that much of what you find is confusing and contradictory.

It seems as though we live in a time of what I call the silent Third World War. What do I mean by this bold statement? The use of pesticides, germicides, fluoride, chlorine, petroleum, genetically modified foods—and God only knows the list of man-made chemicals that have seeped into our air, land and sea—are now out of control. The effect all this poisoning is having on our bodies is incomparable to any other time in history.

There is huge money to be made not only in the pharmaceutical industry but also the "natural" foods, supplements and diet/weight loss industries as well. Everywhere you look there is another product to be sold to cure what ails you. The marketplace is full of schemes, hypes, multi-level networks, gimmicks and gizmos. We are constantly being bombarded with brilliant advertising that convinces us of our need to consume.

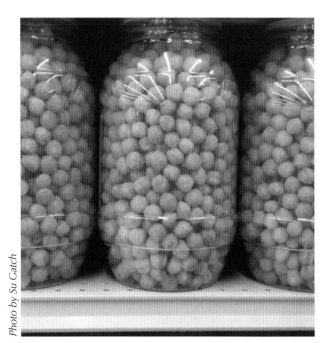

Example of a completely artificial "food product."

All this consumption costs us. It costs us environmentally, socially, politically, physically and spiritually. We look to the world to fix us, save us, rescue us and fulfill us. We bypass the pure goodness that comes to us in nature. We look for the packaged natural remedy or food and forsake God's simple gifts from the garden, hillsides, valleys, farms, forests, lakes, deserts, pastures, vineyards, orchards, streams, lakes and oceans.

When we go out to restaurants, which are commonplace in our fast-paced world, we eat food dripping in rancid oils, over-salted and zapped in microwaves. Most sauces and salad dressings are laden with MSG hidden in deceptive ways. In our frantic pace we look for ways to make life more convenient so we eat denatured, processed, fast and frozen foods. With our constant cultural conditioning to look thin, we attempt all kinds of diets and consume chemicals that we think will cut the corners and cut the fat from our fluffy, bloated, overladen and toxic bodies.

We ingest *excitotoxins*[1] and have no clue what those are and what they really do. We get these excitotoxins in various forms through artificial sweeteners and MSG. MSG is in soup stocks and salad dressings and countless other things you would never imagine. If you try and find it on labels it is insidious. It comes in the veil of nice natural sounding words, like "natural flavoring" or "yeast extract."

Artificial sweeteners are wed with artificial stimulants and made into diet drinks. Everywhere you look in public places there are advertisements encouraging everyone, at any age, to ingest these toxic drinks. Look around at all the soda drinking invitations. They are there to greet you at every gas station, movie theatre, restaurant, airport, airplane, sports events and on and on.

We talk on radioactive phones. We drink bottled water that co-mingles in plastic bottles until it hits your lips. Our city drinking water is contaminated as well as our lakes, streams and oceans. We eat garbage food while we watch garbage television! Our meat, fish and poultry have been exposed to such incredible amounts of poisoning and disease-creating circumstances. It is staggering when you think about the amount of chemicals that bombard and assault us daily.

Photo by Su Gatch

GMO — Man-made Foods

GMOs, or Genetically Modified Organisms, form a major part of the food stream in America. They are being spread around the world in increasing amounts. It is estimated that the average American eats more than their bodyweight in GMOs each year.[2] In addition to the direct consumption of GMO foods, animals in concentrated feeding operations (cattle feedlots, dairies, pig factories, chicken production) are mostly fed GMO grains in the form of GMO corn and soybean.

In the USA, there are no requirements to label GMOs in food products. There have been many attempts at a federal level to legislate this requirement, but powerful corporate interests (Monsanto, etc.) have used their lobby power to block any moves in this direction.

During his campaign for the 2008 presidential election, then-candidate Barack Obama made a speech with an explicit promise saying: "folks ought to have the right to know what is in their food". It was disappointing to see what happened when he took office. Instead of enacting laws to protect the people, he staffed key positions at the Food and Drug Administration and the Department of Agriculture with insiders from Monsanto and the biotech industry.

The November 2012 election in California had a proposition measure on the ballot, which would have required the labeling of GMOs. Had this passed on the state level, it would have probably led to the labeling of GMOs on a national level, as California is a significant part of the total market. The election results were hardly surprising. Before the election campaign began, the polls indicated that over 70% of Californians were in favor of the proposition. However, in the months leading up to the election, a national coalition of big corporate interests that wanted to keep GMOs from being labeled was able to outspend the proposition supporters by a factor of five and blanket California with misleading advertising about the proposition. Due to this advertising, the proposition lost by a few percent. Such is the power of big corporate interests over the food supply in America.

Genetically Modified Organisms are plants or animals that have had segments of DNA from another species artificially implanted which gives traits that are deemed desirable by biotech companies. These are modifications not found in nature, and are not possible through selective breeding or natural selection.

There are two primary ways in which foods are currently genetically modified, although many new modifications are in the works. The first common type of genetic modification is for herbicide resistance. This allows a farmer to drench the field with a potent herbicide such as glyphosate (Roundup) and kill the weeds without harming the crop. The sales pitch is, this will actually reduce the amount of herbicide needed. The second common type of genetic modification is to add a gene that causes plants to produce a Bt toxin, which actually makes the plants toxic to insects. The problem is that this is food that people and animals eat, too!

So far, the most common GMO plants are corn, soybeans, sugar beets, cotton and rape (Canola). However, there are more than 30 different new GMO crops in the pipeline soon to be released. These include alfalfa, salmon (first GMO animal), apples, barley, coffee, carrots, sugar cane, potato and wheat.

When GMO plants are released into the environment they often spread their pollen and contaminate non-GMO crops. When this has happened before, Monsanto has actually sued the farmers whose crops were contaminated!

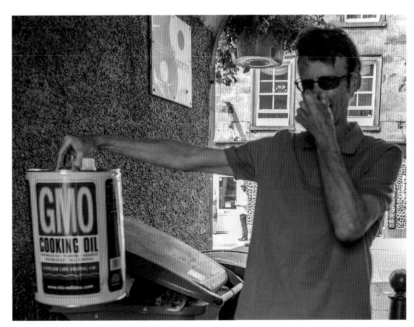

Hell no, we won't GMO!

The herbicide resistance trait is a gold mine for the biotech companies, as they manufacture both the herbicide Roundup and the genetically modified seeds for the crops. Roundup is an herbicide that works by preventing living organisms from being able to absorb certain critical trace minerals such as manganese. This causes plants to get a form of "plant AIDS" and become weakened and die from infection. The herbicide-resistant GMO plants are genetically engineered to have a secondary nutrient pathway so that they can still survive, but they are not as healthy as non-GMO plants and tend to have much lower levels of trace minerals.

There are many side effects to the use of herbicide-resistant GMOs. The use of herbicides has increased by a factor of 10 in the last decade in areas where GMO crops such as corn are common.[3] Significant residues of these herbicides are found in the water, air and food. These powerful herbicides, such as glyphosate, used in ever increasing amounts, have the additional side effect of degrading the soil by harming the natural soil bacteria. This bacterium is what breaks down the organic and inorganic matter in the soil to make it available for the roots of plants to absorb. Consequently, the crops become far less healthy and require even more synthetic fertilizers and other toxic chemicals to kill insects, fungi, etc. that prey upon the weakened plants. Again, this all leads to the plants containing lower levels of nutrients since the soil is not healthy.

The second major type of GMO crop is engineered to create its own toxin, usually the Bt toxin. When we ingest these types of crops, this toxin is in it. Since the introduction of this family of GMO crops, the incidence of Autism and food allergies has skyrocketed.[4] It has been shown that when these foods are eaten, the toxin can be transferred to the natural bacterium that lives in our gut, making it a living pesticide factory.

These GMO foods are imprecise technologies that have many unknown effects on human health. Ranchers who have switched back from GMO feeds to non-GMO feed report that they have far fewer problems with sick animals and fertility problems.[5] The long-term studies to prove the safety of GMOs were never conducted by the FDA in the USA. Biotech companies were able to submit short-term, 3-month feeding studies with rats and conclude that since no problems showed up in the rats after 3 months (the age of adolescence in rats), then GMOs were safe for humans.

An independent study was finally published in France in October 2012, which showed a different, shocking result.[6] When rats were fed diets of GMOs and/or foods with the legally permissible residue levels of glyphosate over a 2-year duration, the horrific results showed high levels of tumors and mortality as compared with the controls. Almost as shocking as the study was Monsanto's immediate reply attacking the study.[7] But, there have been no changes from the government agencies that are responsible for our health.

When rats were fed diets of GMOs and/or foods with legally permissible residue levels of glyphosate... results showed high levels of tumors and mortality compared with the controls.

If you live in America today, the only way to avoid these GMO crops is to buy organic foods or foods that are voluntarily labeled "GMO Free." In Europe, and most of the rest of the world, GMOs are labeled and are not common in foods eaten by people. However, GMOs are still sneaking into the food chain, as GMO animal feeds are used and the resulting meat, dairy and eggs are not labeled. The safest path is to buy organic!

Also found in Europe and incorporated into many bakery and restaurant foods is "vegetable oil" including GMO plants such as rapeseed and soy.

NOTE: Must-have smart phone app: **fooducate.com** (USA only, sorry). This brilliant and timely device will scan the barcodes of everything you could buy and tell you:

◆ What items are GMO

◆ If an item is vegan, vegetarian or organic

◆ Sort out wheat, gluten, food colorings and food allergens

◆ Calorie count and fat content, as well as the good and bad fats

If Man Made It, Don't Eat It

One of my favorite heroes is Jack LaLanne. This amazing man was the godfather of the whole health and fitness movement in the USA. He was teaching people how to eat healthy and exercise long before it was an accepted concept, and he was certainly viewed as a bit of a nut in his early days. He even had one of the first fitness shows on network television, and you can still watch his timeless enthusiasm on YouTube.

Jack worked out for two hours every morning and started his day with freshly made juice. He lived with vital health until he finally succumbed to pneumonia at age 96. According to his family, Jack had worked out the day before he died!

Jack had a favorite saying, "If man made it, don't eat it". This so perfectly summarizes what you need to do in order to eat a healthy diet. Somehow, people tend to polarize into different diet camps…. The Paleos, Vegans, Raws, Low GI, Gluten Free, Vegetarian, Pescetarianism, low fat, low carb, high protein, etc. However, when you look at different cultures and how people have thrived for thousands of years all over the globe, it becomes clear that we are omnivores, and can subsist on a wide variety of different diets. For example, Inuit eat a diet with far more animal products and fat than natives of Central America. What all traditional cultures have in common is eating a local diet, not processed in a food factory, made up of whole, natural food, containing an abundance of phytochemicals and natural macro and micronutrients.

Over thousands of years of relative geographic isolation, while eating the local diet, there was a natural selection forcing function in which people with metabolisms that thrived on the locally available natural diet were the ones who survived, reproduced the most and passed on their own genes. For example, today we see that some people can tolerate lactose and others cannot. Some people's bodies can tolerate more fats and cholesterol than others.

Fortunately, there has been some interesting research on the diet and average lifespans of a few different specific cultures that lead the world in healthy aging. In the article "Secrets of Living Longer" by Dan Buettner in the November 2005 issue of *National Geographic,* Buettner examines populations from three different areas and cultures: modern 7th Day Adventists from Loma Linda, California; villagers from traditional cultures in Okinawa, Japan; and people from the highlands of Sardinia, Italy. These populations are noted for having more than twice as many people living past 100 than the normal population, and much lower rates of degenerative diseases of old age. No fad diets here, just some common sense principles for eating and living.

What were the common elements in these three different cultures? Spending time with family and friends, constant moderate physical activity, no smoking and a plant-based diet with legumes. Interestingly, the 7th Day Adventists and Okinawans both abstained from alcohol, while the Sardinians enjoyed red wine, with its high polyphenol content. In a subsequent study of the long-living inhabitants of the Greek Island Ikaria, Buettner observed the same emphasis on social time with family and friends along with constant moderate physical activity.[8] But their diet included more animal products. The average Ikarian ate fish twice a week, meat five times a month and goat's milk several times per week. They also consumed a large amount of unheated olive oil and two to four glasses of wine a day.

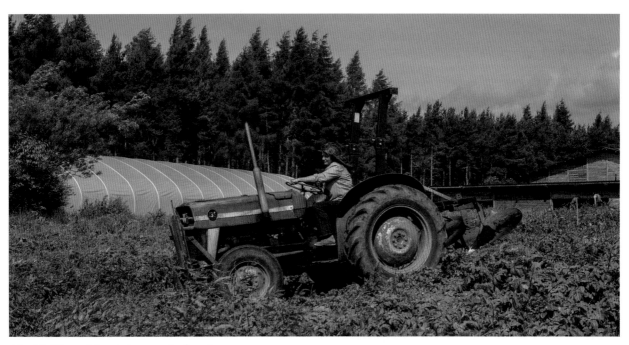

No GMO on Maggie's organic farm!

Obviously, diet does have a significant impact on health and longevity. None of the long-living populations in these studies ate a diet that was anywhere close to the Standard American Diet. Fast foods, feedlot-farmed, hormone-laced meat and highly processed factory food, are not eaten by these people who live longer than the rest of us. They simply eat mostly vegetables and a natural pure diet of unprocessed, unfractionated foods with high nutrient density. Eating healthy is really quite simple. It only gets complicated when you try to fit man-made foods into the equation. Keep life simple and remember: "If man made it, don't eat it".

Manufactured Food

I sometimes feel as if I am constantly falling down the rabbit hole with this whole process of trying to eat a healthy diet. Things are sometimes just not what they seem, and recently I just had a new awareness that is going to be radically changing how I approach eating from now on. The bottom line, I have had to relearn the truth of Jack LaLanne's brilliant quote: "If man made don't eat it".

What I have recently learned again is that any processed food made in a factory is highly suspect. Robyn and I are both very aware of what we eat, and try to eat a very pure diet with limited refined or processed foods. We choose organic whenever possible, eat lots of raw veggies and fruit, and limit the amount of animal products we eat. For various reasons we choose to eat some animal products, but choose quality over quantity and only organic and grass fed.

Last week I took a close look at the fine print of the ingredient lists of a few manufactured food items that we have been regularly eating and asked myself "What is that, really"? In the process of doing this, I have developed a new appreciation for the need to be vigilant and suspicious when it comes to eating anything that comes in a package or has a bar code. If it is processed in a factory with an ingredient list and a product name, then it is manufactured under the rules of capitalism.

The Rules of Capitalism Are Not
The Rules of Health

When a food is manufactured in a factory for sale and profit, it means that someone else, and not you, is making the decisions about what ingredients to add to the food you will be putting into your body. These decisions are not based on what is healthy for you, but rather what will make the most profit for the manufacturing company. Don't kid yourself, they may have a corporate spokesman or logo of a happy chef, smiling housewife or contented child, but this is all an elaborate front. The reality of manufactured food is, the ingredients are selected to make the food taste better (so they will sell more) and be the lowest cost possible with best shelf life in order to maximize the profit margins for the manufacturers and distribution chain. If you are trying to eat a healthy, pure diet, please remember the food industry's needs and interests are not the same as yours.

I don't have a jar of tri-calcium phosphate in my spice cupboard or anywhere in my kitchen. Do you?

Surprises in the Pantry

We like to have green smoothies in the morning for breakfast. This is a great way to have a high nutrient density meal to start the day. I like to add lots of raw veggies such as kale or spinach and green powders such as spirulina. For the liquid, I had been using a store-bought almond milk, thinking this would be a healthy non-dairy alternative.

Last week we returned from the store with 10 litres of almond milk, since they were on sale. This stack of containers dominated the floor of my pantry and I thought to myself: "Hmm, we really look like heavy users of this particular product." Indeed we were, since we drank a good amount each morning. At that point, I thought it would be a good idea to take a closer look at the label.

Sure enough, there was an ingredient in this almond milk that was highly suspicious. In order to make the "calcium" claim on the packaging, to boost sales and to help emulsify the liquid mixture, the manufacturer had added tri-calcium phosphate. I don't know what naturally contains tri-calcium phosphate, but this didn't sound like a substance that should be added to my food. After all, I don't have a jar of tri-calcium phosphate in my spice cupboard or anywhere in my kitchen. Do you? Perhaps my mother has an old dusty jar of it in the corner of her garage; a long lost relic from my boyhood chemistry set.

Tri-calcium phosphate stood out on the almond milk label because I had recently read an article in a German Medical Journal *Deutsches Ärzteblatt International* about the health risks from phosphate additives in food.[9] In this article, the researchers demonstrate that the addition of inorganic phosphates to processed foods increases the risks of cardiovascular disease and kidney damage. Why should I needlessly take this risk so that a food manufacturer can make more money?

After that, we found a different brand of almond milk with no tri-calcium phosphate. I should have read the label more closely in the store. A closer examination of the label at home revealed that it contained a different emulsifier, carrageenan. Although it is derived from seaweed and therefore appears to be safe and natural, it turns out that carrageenan is not benign. In an article in *Environmental Health Perspectives*[10], researchers demonstrate that there is an association between exposure to carrageenan and the occurrence of colonic ulcerations and gastrointestinal abnormal growths in animals. The researchers also recommended that because of the possible inflammatory bowel disease and colon cancer promoting effects of carrageenan, the widespread use of carrageenan in the western diet should be reconsidered.

The man-made food story keeps going… I also realized that the organic, commercial soup broth powders (sold in health food stores) I had been using contained large amounts of MSG. This is cleverly disguised as "yeast extract". I had been regularly eating large amounts of an excitotoxin without even knowing it. You can read more about it when we talk about real soup broths.

Buyer Beware

The message here is clear: Whenever you eat food that has been processed you take the risk of eating impure food. Manufactured food is designed to increase sales, not benefit your health. These are not isolated incidences. Tri-calcium phosphate, carrageenan and yeast extract are found in many different processed foods. They are considered normal in the modern, man-made western diet. And, these particular additives are just the tip of the manufactured food additive iceberg! Please take the time to read the label. If it contains any ingredients that you don't have on your kitchen shelf or your grandmother wouldn't recognize, then ask some questions and do some research. The answers may shock you.

Numbered references — see page 176.

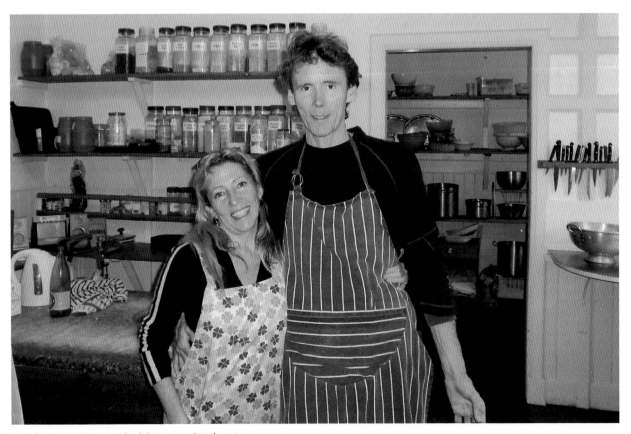

Cooking in the Newbold House kitchen!

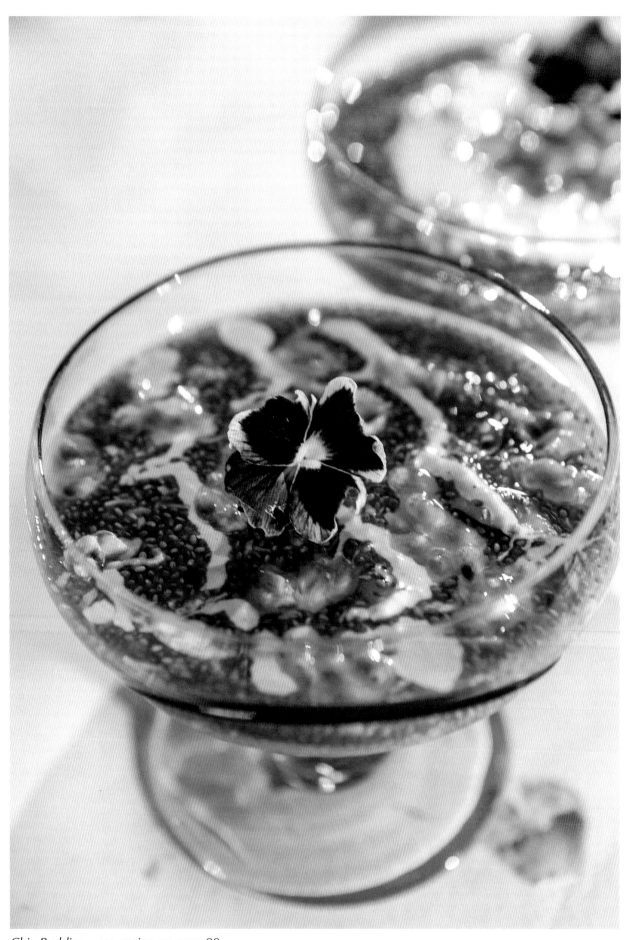

Chia Pudding – see recipe on page 99.

14

CHAPTER 2
How, What, and Where to Get PURE Foods

PURE Foods are Essential, and Stand For:

Phytonutrients
Unprocessed
Raw and
Enzyme-rich

As advocates for eating PURE foods, we are passionate about saying that no matter what you decide is best for your body (whether that be eating as a carnivore, vegetarian, vegan, raw foodist or paleo), it is essential to eat a balance of high nutrient dense foods, grown organically, unprocessed, with as many enzymes intact as possible. If you intuitively feel best being all raw, vegan or mostly raw, then you must take care to understand why and how to get the balance of nutrients it takes for your body to thrive on. Without including at least a small amount of quality animal products, it can be challenging, over time to be able to get enough vitamin B and iron. Not to say it is impossible. Different bodies respond differently. Make your priority finding what truly works best for your optimal health.

It is not our intention to tell people one way to eat. When we look through the magical lens of hyperspace and learn about the world at large, both past and present, we see a range of interesting conclusions about food. Certainly many studies can support the exclusion of animal products and point to people who have thrived from doing this. For some, (certainly not the majority) eating all raw, vegan is healthier for them as individuals, not because they are healthier in general. However, statistically, a total absence of animal products reveals that underlying deficiencies tend to surface over time.[11]

The Weston A. Price Foundation and one of our favorite authors, Sally Fallon (who wrote *Nourishing Traditions*) have wonderful information in regards to the value of eating grass fed, free range animal proteins and fats, especially for generations of indigenous people all over the world throughout history.[12]

Certain facts are undeniable. For eons, humans evolved eating diets including animal foods and fats. Through generational inheritance, humans became accustomed to, and able to function well on, these foods. However, what was absent over generations of time was processed grains, carbohydrates, and sugars. Herein lies the root of our current inflammatory diseases.

Ethnic and racial backgrounds are important factors to consider when you tap into what is intuitively best for you. Intuitive eating is linked to wise thinking. The two go hand and hand. True intuitive thinking will lead you to the truth for your unique needs. The way you will know is by how you feel (mood, energy, bowel regularity, vitality, etc.), as well as the results you get over time.

P Is for Phytochemicals

Phytochemicals are substances found in foods and are comprised of natural chemicals with protective or disease preventive properties. Unlike carbohydrates, proteins and fats, phytochemicals are considered nonessential nutrients, as they are not required for sustaining life. It has been well understood that in nature, phytochemicals help plants to protect themselves from the ravages of pests, harmful chemicals and diseases. Current research suggests phytochemicals also provide great benefits to humans, especially as prevention and protection towards common diseases. Scientists are aware of well over a thousand known phytochemicals. Some of the more commonly known phytochemicals that you might be aware of are lycopene in tomatoes, isoflavones in soy and flavonoids in fruit.

What do phytochemicals do?

Phytochemicals found in our foods can vary and produce a range of beneficial actions and effects. Let's take a look at examples of specific foods that contain powerful phytochemicals, creating health promoting results.[13]

Anti-bacterial effect – Garlic contains the phytochemical allicin.

Antioxidant – Onions, leeks, and garlic contain allyl sulfides; fruits and carrots contain carotenoids; fruits and vegetables have flavonoids; and tea, as well as grapes, contain polyphenols. Most phytochemicals contain antioxidant properties, some more than others. Antioxidants help to scavenge free radicals and protect our cells against oxidative stress. This reduces the risk of certain types of cancer.

Hormonal action – Soy contains isoflavones, which can imitate human estrogens. This aids in the reduction of menopausal symptoms and osteoporosis.

Interference with DNA replication – Beans have saponins that interfere with the replication of cell DNA, thus preventing cancer cells from multiplying. Hot peppers contain the phytochemical capsaicin that protects DNA from carcinogens.

Stimulation of enzymes – Cabbages contains phytochemicals thought to help lower the risk of breast cancer. These phytochemicals, known as indoles, help stimulate enzymes that lessen the effects of estrogen. Other phytochemicals with similar effects are protease inhibitors found in soy and beans, and terpenes found in citrus fruits and cherries.

Physical action – Cranberries contain proanthocyanidins with the amazing ability to bind physically to cell walls, thereby preventing the adhesion of pathogens to human cell walls.

How Do We Get Enough Phytochemicals?

Most foods contain some phytochemicals, some more than others. The easiest way to get more phytochemicals is to eat more fruit (blueberries, cranberries, cherries, apples...) and vegetables (cauliflower, cabbage, carrots, broccoli, kale, spinach...). The recommended daily amount is 5 to 9 servings of fruits or vegetable. Fruits and vegetables are also rich in minerals, vitamins and fiber and low in saturated fat.

To ensure anywhere from 3–6 servings of antioxidants, start your day by making a high nutrient dense smoothie, (like the one we suggest in this book). Eating foods rich in phytochemicals in their raw form helps to preserve the enzymes. Simply put, the more enzymes, the more life. The more you increase your intake of phytochemicals, especially ones which contain antioxidants and are enzyme rich (foods not heated past 118°F or 47°C), the more you provide your body with nutrients that will feed you on a cellular level, help to slow the aging process and provide cancer-prevention potential.

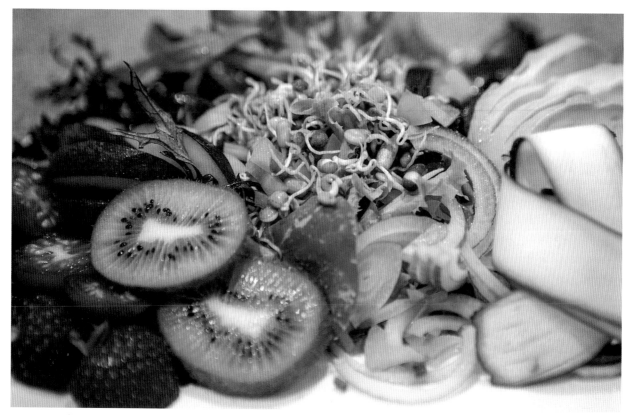

A range of fresh fruits and vegetables, prepared by Intuitive Chef Wendy at Rockvilla Restaurant and B&B, Lochcarron, Scotland

Foods and Plants Containing Phenomenal Phytochemicals

Fruit, Vegetables and Nuts:

Acai	Broccoli	Cranberry	Olive	Sweet Potatoes
Almond	Brussel Sprouts	Grape	Orange	Strawberries
Beets	Cabbage	Hazelnut	Pomegranate	Tomatoes
Bilberry	Cantaloupe	Kale	Potatoes	Wolfberry
Blackberry	Carrots	Lettuce	Red Peppers	Yams
Blackcurrant	Cauliflower	Mangos	Red Raspberry	
Black Raspberry	Celery	Noni	Soybeans	
Blueberry	Corn	Nuts	Spinach	

NOTE: dark-colored fruits and vegetables have more antioxidants than other fruits and vegetables.

Beans and Seeds:

Cocoa	Flaxseeds	Soy

Medicinal Plants:

Comfrey	Goat's Rue	Opium Poppy	Red Bryony
Common Broom	Lesser Celandine	Passion Fruit	Valerian
Echinacea Ginkgo	Lungwort	Periwinkle	Wintergreen

Common Herbs:

Aloe Vera	Dandelion	Korean Ginseng	Red Clover	Sweet Clover
American Ginseng	Ground Ivy	Lemon Balm	Rooibos	Tea
Clary Sage	Hawthorn	Lemon Verbena	Rosemary	Wild Carrot
Common Mallow	Hop	Marigold	Sage	Wild Pansy
Common Yarrow	Hyssop	Milk Thistle	Schizandra	Woodruff
Cornsilk	Indian Cress	Oregano	Stinging Nettle	

U Is for Unprocessed

Food-like substances sold as "food" are found in rows and rows of assorted flavors and sizes. GMO corn and corn syrup are the underpinnings of thousands of products. Never underestimate the power of dyes in foods.

Why eat whole, unprocessed, organic foods? Because that is the way they come to us in nature and because the sum of an object is greater than its lesser parts. The elements that make up a piece of fruit for example, work together synergistically. A good example of this is an orange, having the bioflavonoids contained in the membranous whitish skin. If we denature food, then we leave out elements that create a complete or whole nutritional package intended as nourishment for our bodies.

When we take milk and pasteurize it or homogenize it, we now have a different food. The nutrient value changes dramatically and ends up costing our body the ability to assimilate and digest it in this altered form. Foods that have been altered or used in part are known as fractionated foods.

Optimally, it is best to get foods organic and as freshly picked as is possible. Of whole foods, the absolute best are those foods that are still living. Living foods mean they are still alive and growing. Once you pick an apple off the tree, it is no longer connected to the source that courses through it to make it continue to grow. It will not get any larger once off the branch. Sunflower sprouts, in contrast, are a living food. They are still thriving when you pop them in your mouth, as long as they haven't sat around too long.

For people who include animal products, be sure to always buy organic, as chemicals bond to fats. Also make sure animal products are hormone- and antibiotic-free. Always choose wild, free range or grass fed, whenever possible. You will hear us say this countless times throughout the book. This message needs to spread far and wide!

Upgrade to Unprocessed Whole Foods

Think of this change as a chance to find new and better things

Replace Processed	Embrace Unprocessed
White sugar	Dates, honey, maple syrup
White rice	Brown rice, quinoa
Cow's milk	Raw goat milk, almond milk, coconut milk
Regular eggs	Organic, free-range, pastured eggs
Canned foods/frozen food	Fresh fruit and vegetables
Processed oils, canola/rapeseed oil	Olive oil, coconut oil, organic butter, Udo's Choice Oil Blend
Table salt	Himalayan salt
Yogurts with sugar added	Plain (goat) yogurt; add your own fruit or fruit juice sweetened jam

Embracing the New

If eating healthier is new for you, each time you go shopping, replace old items with new and healthier versions. For some it is a question of tightening up the loose edges. One of the first items we recommend that you buy would be canning jars with screw tight lids. Storing your staples in glass jars is a wonderful way to prolong the shelf life of your food.

We use large (3 litres) jars for surplus bulk items like nuts, grains, and legumes. Spices can be stored in small glass jars. Get veggies out of plastic bags and into glass pyrex containers with lids or BPA free, Lock & Lock containers to neatly store and stack. You can see how tidy it keeps the fridge and makes it easy to see and get exactly what you need. We use glass jars to store our dry goods, broths or batches of fresh juice.

We also use jars to store our dehydrated raw flax/linseed and chia crackers and soaked and sprouted, then dehydrated nuts and seeds. This is the best way to keep these great raw snacks fresh and handy.

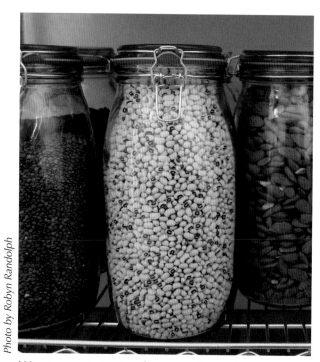

Photo by Robyn Randolph

We use quart size jars for our daily staples.

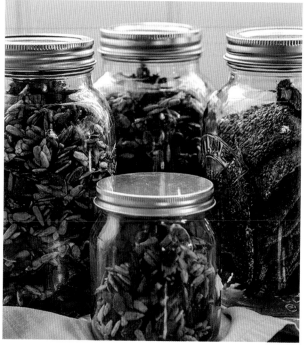

Jars are also the way to keep dehydrated snacks fresh.

PURE Shopping!

You can begin by buying any or all of the following staples. Replace your old canned foods with a variety of brightly colored whole foods and store them in airtight jars that can be found on **amazon.com**.

Fresh Staples:

Can be stored or displayed in baskets on countertops or in containers in fridge.

Apples
Apricots
Asparagus
Artichokes
Aubergine
Avocados
Bananas
Beet greens
Beets
Berries
   (all kinds)
Bok Choy
Broccoli
Brussels
   sprouts
Cabbage
Carrots
Cauliflower
Celeriac
Celery
Chard
Cherries
Chives
Coconuts
Collards
Courgette

Cucumbers
Dandelion
   greens
Dates
Eggplant
Eggs
Endive
Fennel
Fresh herbs:
   Basil
   Coriander
   Dill
   Parsley
   Rosemary
   Sage
   Thyme
   Turmeric
Garlic
Ginger
Grapefruit
Grapes
Kale
Kiwi
Kohlrabi
Kumquats
Lemons
Lettuce

Limes
Mangos
Melons
Mushrooms
Nectarines
Onions
Oranges
Papayas
Peaches
Pears
Peas
Peppers
Pineapple
Pumpkin
Rhubarb
Satsumas
Spinach
Squash
Sweet
   potatoes
Tomatoes
Turnips
Watercress
Yams
Zucchini

NOTE: Store fresh herbs in airtight containers in the fridge and buy as required for specific recipes.

Dried Fruits

Apricots
Shredded
   coconut
Currants

Papaya
Persimmons
Prunes

Raisins
Sun-dried
   tomatoes

NOTE: Due to high-carbohydrate levels affecting blood sugar, use these sparingly: bananas, beets, carrots, eggplant, jicama, winter squashes, yams and sweet potatoes. Best to omit all potatoes.

Grains:

Brown rice, Oat groats, Quinoa

These are the only ones we suggest, and should be used sparingly, along with good fats and proteins.

Legumes:

Black-eyed peas
Yellow split peas
Black beans
Garbanzo beans

Kidney beans
Dried green peas
Lentils
Pinto beans

Nuts and Seeds:

Almonds
Cashews
Chia seeds
Flaxseeds
Hazelnuts

Linseeds
Macadamia
   nuts
Pecans
Pumpkin
   seeds

Sesame seeds
Sunflower
   seeds
Walnuts

Herbs, Spices and Oils:

Basil
Bay leaves
Black pepper
Cajun spice
Carob powder
Cayenne
Chili pepper
   flakes
Chipotle
   powder
Cilantro
Cinnamon
Cumin
   powder
Curry powder
Dill

Fresh garlic
Garlic powder
Fresh ginger
Ginger
   powder
Himalayan salt
Italian
   seasoning
Lemongrass
Marjoram
Nutmeg
Onion flakes
Onion
   powder
Oregano
Paprika

Parsley
Pumpkin spice
Red pepper
   flakes
Rosemary
Thyme
Turmeric
Vanilla bean

Organic
   coconut oil
Organic
   olive oil
Krill oil
Udo's oil

Other Staples:

Almond butter (raw)
Apple cider vinegar
Apricot jam
   (unsweetened)
Balsamic vinegar
Barley grass
Brown rice vinegar
Butter (organic)
Capers
Chlorella
Cook's vanilla
Carob powder
Cocoa powder (raw)
Date syrup

Goat yogurt and
   homemade whey
Honey or
   Manuka honey
Meats and poultry,
   (organic, grass-fed)
   for non-vegans
Miso paste
Nama shoyu or wheat-
   free shoyu/tamari
Tahini (raw)
Sauerkraut (raw)
Spirulina

How much money do you spend on coffee and alcohol? How much do you spend on going out to eat? Start with eliminating those things and see how much money you have.

Start with what you can afford. Fats are the first priority when buying organic food on a limited budget. Most people assume the first place to spend for organic food is on fruits and vegetables. Throughout the book you will hear us repeat over and over again…*chemicals bond to fats, therefore buy all your fats organic first (includes: oil, nuts, seeds, and all animal products).*

Top 10 PURE Revival foods:

1. **Spirulina would be the one thing I would suggest getting first, for these reasons:**

   ◆ It is a complete whole food. You could live on it if you had to.

   ◆ Powdered spirulina can easily be mixed into liquids.

   ◆ Great survival food and good to have for emergencies.

   ◆ No special equipment needed.

   ◆ Cost per nutritional value, excellent investment in nourishing yourself.

   ◆ Spirulina is an immune system builder, detoxifier, and blood purifier.

   ◆ It has a very long shelf life without using any preservatives or additives.

   ◆ A great way to alkalize.

2. **Organic Pastured Eggs**: relatively inexpensive for high-quality nutritional benefits, especially quality protein and fat. A great source of naturally occurring B12, lutein (antioxidant important for eyes), choline (brain, nervous and cardiovascular health). Best to eat eggs as close to raw as possible. Can throw into smoothies (give it a whirl)! I like to boil water, quickly dip the egg in the boiled water and then rinse it off to clean it before opening it.

3. **Kale** – in our opinion, King of Vegetables! It is a cruciferous vegetable loaded with phytonutrients, vitamins A, B, and C as well a great source of calcium, iron, indole-3-carbinol (recommended for colon cancer prevention).

4. **Nuts** – raw almonds and walnuts are the two top nuts we recommend, as both are rich in phytochemicals. Almonds are a great source of vitamin E as well as magnesium, calcium, potassium, and phosphorus. Almonds are a good vegan protein as well. Walnuts supply great omega-3 fats and are essential for vegans.

5. **Avocados** are a fantastic food for young and old. Loaded with phytochemicals and especially rich in healthy fats as well as vitamin E, B, potassium

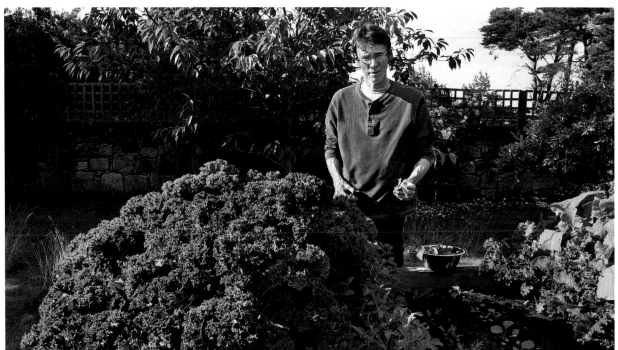

Photo by Robyn Randolph

Kale is "The King of Vegetables," in our opinion!

and folic acid. A wonderful food to replace grain carbohydrates. Fuel food at its best!

6. **Wild salmon from uncontaminated waters** (Alaskan). Excellent source of omega-3 fats, high antioxidant value, and great quality protein.

7. **Organic coconut oil** contains a rare natural fat called lauric acid. This fat is a medium chain triglyceride, not stored in the body like other fats, but used immediately for fuel and energy. Lauric acid provides anti-viral, anti-bacterial and anti-microbial properties. The health benefits now being studied and promoted from the saturated fats in coconut oil include promoting heart health, weight loss, immune system health, supporting a healthy metabolism, great benefits for diabetics, MS, Parkinson's, some cancers and most recently, Alzheimer's and dementia prevention.

8. **Raw organic grass-fed butter** is the best form of vitamin A, especially for kids. Butter contains short and medium chain fats, supporting immune function. Butter also contains important trace minerals and antioxidants.

9. **Fresh juice with spinach, kale, carrots, celery, and ginger** is a great way to pack in phytonutrients and high density nutrition. If you have a limited budget and can't afford a good juicer, treat yourself to a fresh juice at a juice bar instead of going out to coffee.

10. **Blueberries** are power-packed with phytochemicals and could very well be the Queen of Fruit! If you wed blueberries with kale once a day… what a dynamic duo you would have reigning in you! High in natural fiber and low in sugar so you can keep your blood sugar balanced, blueberries are a great snack or on-the-go food and great for kids. Just mix blueberries in a bowl, with cinnamon and a little vanilla. Easy and yum!

You'll find lots more info on our websites, including our top 30 nutrient-dense foods to stock up on, and an A-to-Z list of PURE whole foods and their nutrient values. (These can be found under the blog-archive posts link.)

NOTE: We like all our foods as close to whole, fresh, local, and organic as possible. However, there are a few PURE, organic, whole-food "supplements" that we find extremely beneficial. We consider these whole food supplements as immune-building and vitality-sustaining staples.

We distribute several of these and some of our very favorite PURE foods, as people often ask us how they can get the superfoods we recommend. Our intent is to be helpful and provide resources for PURE foods and quality equipment. Check our websites for updates, free recipes, and current sources. Please contact us if you have any questions:

purehighlandliving.com (UK/USA)
phporder.com/rawsome (USA)

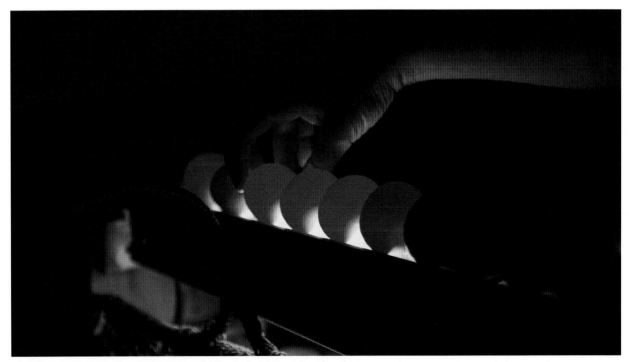

Grading eggs at Laikenbuie Organic Farm in Nairn, Scotland

Our Favorite PURE Superfoods

Barley grass is a wonderful way for vegetarians to get all essential amino acids. Amino acids are the building blocks of proteins, which are the major components of every cell in the body. Barley grass contains polypeptides, which are smaller proteins, making them more easily absorbed directly into the bloodstream where they promote cell metabolism. Loaded with valuable enzymes and a wide spectrum of vitamins and minerals, barley grass powder becomes a whole food concentrate. Please note that barley grass powder is made from the green grass, not the mature seed head, which is the grain barley. Therefore, barley grass is completely gluten free and has none of the adverse issues associated with grains. (See Chapter 6, *Get Equipped* for how to order.)

The chlorophyll in this grass is as close to human hemoglobin as is found in nature. Chlorophyll's benefits are numerous but one that is quite impressive according to an article in the *Journal of the National Cancer Institute* (Jan. 4, 1995) states that chlorophyll fed to laboratory animals was found to reduce absorption of three dietary carcinogens. This is an excellent way to help maintain a healthy acid-alkaline balance essential in preventing many diseases. Barley grass coupled with raw vegetable juicing (especially carrot) is one of the best superfoods, with great benefits for patients recovering from cancer.

Bee pollen is a wonderful complement to sprinkle on top of smoothies or you can just eat a heaping teaspoon in the morning. This is a wonderful way to get your B-complex vitamins, essential during stressful times. Bee pollen is an immune strengthener loaded with vitamins, amino acids, essential fatty acids and minerals and is comprised of approximately 15% protein. In weight-loss programs, bee pollen has been suggested for its ability to stimulate the metabolic processes. It contains 15% lecithin by volume. Lecithin is a substance that helps dissolve and flush fat from the body and helps to lower low-density lipoproteins (LDL) while increasing the helpful high-density lipoproteins (HDL). Some people are allergic to bee pollen so it is best to start out with a very small amount like 1/8 of a teaspoon. Then, work up slowly to about 1 teaspoon, watching for any reactions.

Fresh carrot juice is a must do if you own a juicer. When possible we recommend making fresh juice on your "2 days." Adding barley grass powder to fresh carrot juice bumps up the phytochemical and nutrient density to a wonderful wholesome level. You will love the pairing of these two together. Drinking barley grass on its own is a bit like drinking a freshly mowed lawn. I suppose if you were a cow that would make you salivate! Mixed in carrot juice, barley grass comes alive, bursting with nutrients in a palate-pleasing way. Carrot-barley juice is another great way to get important minerals, which is becoming harder to do as our soils are more and more depleted. When you shop for the week, make sure you always have a good supply of carrots on hand for juicing.

Chia seeds are native to South America and have been a staple for centuries. They are tiny little

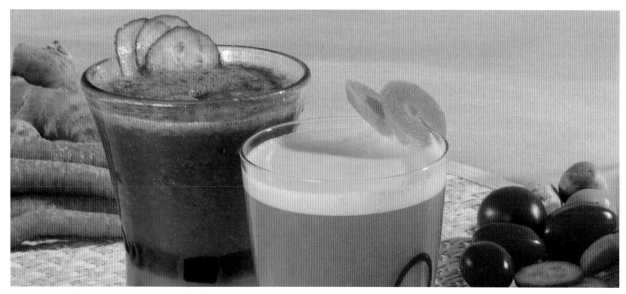

Adding barley grass powder to fresh carrot juice bumps up the phytochemical and nutrient density to a wonderful wholesome level.

seeds looking much like poppy seeds, loaded with nutrients and antioxidants. Chia seeds are one of the richest plant based sources of omega-3 fatty acids (specifically, alpha-linolenic acid, or ALA), known to help reduce inflammation, reduce cholesterol and enhance cognitive performance. They can play an important role in blood sugar regulation helping to reduce insulin resistance. Gluten and grain free, we highly recommend adding them as much as possible into your daily diet. When soaked, the seeds become gelatinous and can be used as an egg replacer for binding ingredients together. Chia seeds are great to throw in smoothies, good for making raw crackers or use for making "porridge" or "pudding". See Coconut Chia Pineapple Passion Porridge/Pudding. Chia seeds can be found at most health food stores.

Chlorella is nature's richest food source of chlorophyll, a powerful cleanser and detoxifier. Japan's #1 supplement, commonly recommended to aid the body in the elimination of heavy metals and other toxins such as DDT, mercury, cadmium and lead.

Chlorella has been found to enhance immunity, increasing production of the antiviral, anticancer immune factor, interferon, as well as the activity of T cells and macrophages against viral invaders and cancer cells. Its well-documented cleansing effects in the liver are believed to further support the body's natural resistance against diseases, including those caused by viruses. Natural killer cell activity has also been found to improve with chlorella supplementation—a suggestion that this algae could protect against the secondary bacterial infections that often occur in the wake of colds and flu. Supplements of a high-molecular weight fraction of Chlorella pyrenoidosa were found to boost antibody response to influenza vaccinations in people aged 55 and younger, improving subjects' response to the vaccines and better protecting them against contracting the flu.

One of the most promising aspects of chlorella is a unique chemical it contains called Chlorella Growth Factor (CGF). Within the plant itself, CGF is responsible for controlling cell division and growth, which occurs with amazing rapidity, increasing its biomass four times every 20 to 24 hours. Lab mice fed CGF enjoy increases in life span of over 30%. Chlorella is the fastest-

replicating single-cell organism and CGF protects cells when they are most vulnerable to mutation, during replication.

Coconut oil is being crowned as one of the world's most beneficial whole foods and oils. Research has proven that the fat content of coconuts is made up primarily of medium-chain triglycerides, which are used immediately in the body as an energy source. This type of fat does not circulate in the blood stream leading to weight gain and other health problems. Studies indicate effectiveness against parasites, fungus and viruses. Great benefits, such as preventing osteoporosis, improving digestion and nutrient absorption are heralded. Coconut oil is marvellous for keeping the skin soft and smooth, and may help prevent premature aging and wrinkles. The most exciting new area of study is coconut oils ability to affect the brain and potentially aid and prevent Alzheimer's.

Essential fats (the good, the bad and the ugly!)

Let's start with the ugly fats—hydrogenated fats like margarine and shortening are the worst and can cause heart disease. Chemically fried fats are known as junk fats and can be seen on package labels as "partially hydrogenated" or "hydrogenated" and are found in most cookies and crackers. These oils have been fried with hydrogen along with metal catalysts (used to help flip the carbon chain around by 180 degrees to a trans configuration) for prolonged periods of time. The purpose of this is to change them from their natural liquid state into solid trans-fats. These types of fats will absolutely lead to heart disease, as the body cannot process them properly. The inevitable buildup on the arterial walls seriously impairs the blood flow.

Prior to the introduction of seed oils at the turn of the 20th century, heart disease was rare. Also around that time, margarine was introduced into the marketplace as a less expensive alternative. By the mid-20th century margarine overtook butter in popularity. Over time, people became convinced that butter was a bad fat and margarine and seed oils were better.[14]

Buried information is finally beginning to surface. A recent article we read in the *British Science Journal* only weeks ago debunked the common belief that the use of animal fats is bad and the use

> *The most exciting new area of study is coconut oil's ability to affect the brain and potentially aid and prevent Alzheimer's.*

of vegetable oil is good. According to the journal, scientists and doctors are finally coming to a new conclusion based on the importance of getting the right balance of the essential omega-3 and omega-6 fats. Not only is the right ratio (1:1) of these oils important but the quality and integrity of the oils are as well. When omega-6 oils are oxidized or become rancid, these oils become hazardous to our health. Omega-6 oils are in abundance in the typical processed food chain, whereas quality omega-3 oils are often left out. This lopsided balance of eating too much damaged omega-6 oil and not enough quality (non rancid or oxidized) omega-3 oil sets the body up for disease in the form of cardiovascular disease, cancer, Alzheimer's, rheumatoid arthritis, and diabetes.[15]

Important steps to ensure the proper balance of omega-3 to omega-6 fats

1. Reduce omega-6; avoid all processed foods and foods cooked at high temperature in vegetable oils.
2. Increase use of heart-healthy omega-3 fats (krill oil, spirulina, chlorella, Udo's oil, flaxseeds/linseed, walnuts)

The truth about butter

Butter is a saturated fat that can actually help lower triglycerides. Did you know that butter is the best and most easily absorbed source of vitamin A? It also contains the antioxidants selenium and vitamin E. You just can't beat the quality of the vitamin A that butter provides, which is essential for promoting healthy growth in children.[16] (Be sure to only use organic.)

We believe the absolute best source of butter is when it is clarified through heating and becomes

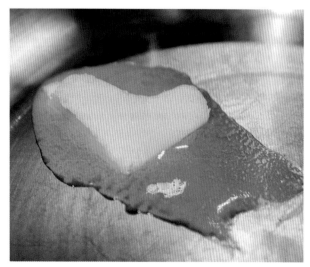

It's ok to LOVE butter and use plenty of it. Organic butter is a great healthy fat!

ghee. Check on YouTube for videos showing how to make homemade ghee.

Essential fatty acids are essential; hence we need quality fat on a regular basis:

◆ For the production of all hormones

◆ To protect our internal organs

◆ To burn for fuel when food is not readily available

◆ To help maintain our sex drive

◆ To maintain mental clarity

◆ To avoid carbohydrate cravings

◆ To keep our bowels working properly

◆ To help some women avoid fertility problems

◆ To act as barriers in our cells to keep out harmful microbes

◆ To maintain healthy hair, skin and to combat eczema

◆ To help support neuron connections vital in brain's communication system

◆ Because nerve, brain, eye, heart, adrenal and thyroid cells require essential fats to function

◆ Because fat is necessary for the production of serotonin, which is key in elevating mood and promoting sleep

◆ To maintain healthy heart and arteries

◆ To treat diabetic neuropathy

◆ To relieve PMS and cyclical breast pain

◆ To prevent gallstones

◆ Because it will actually help with weight loss (omega-3 fats raise our metabolic rate and act as diuretics, helping kidneys flush excess water from tissues)

Some food sources of omega-3 fats are: fish and shellfish, eggs, grass-fed beef, flaxseed (linseed), hemp oil, chia seeds, pumpkin seeds, sunflower seeds, leafy vegetables and walnuts.

Good supplement choices for essential fats are krill oil and Udo's Choice Blend (for vegetarians/ vegans), also discussed in this section.

The best fats to use for cooking are organic butter and coconut oil. Olive oil is a wonderful fat. However, it is NOT a good oil for high temperature cooking.

TIP: Try using coconut oil instead of butter. Or use a blend of coconut oil and butter. Also add coconut oil or Udo's Oil to fruit smoothies to slow down the intake of the sugar. This will make it easier on the pancreas to process and will help keep blood sugar levels a little more even.

The best healthy fats for your daily diet are: coconut oil, olive oil, olives, butter, eggs, Udo's oil, fish oils, avocados and nuts. As chemicals bond to fats, be sure to always buy your fats organic.

Fermented foods – traditionally lacto-fermented foods are an ancient food preservation technique, produced through the breakdown of carbohydrates and proteins by microorganisms such as bacteria, yeast and molds. Also known as "functional foods", they are extremely beneficial to overall health and in particular to our gut health, being considered a form of probiotic. Eating foods prepared in the traditional lacto-fermented way — such as olives, pickles, yogurt and sauerkraut — helps to promote the growth of friendly intestinal bacteria. This is essential, given the condition of our gut health from the foods we have ingested in this modern culture. They say health begins in the gut. Additionally these foods increase B vitamins (even the hard-to-get vitamin B12 (a must for vegans and raw foodies), omega-3 fatty acids, digestive enzymes, lactase and lactic acid and other immune chemicals that fight off harmful bacteria and certain cancer cells.[17]

Flaxseeds/linseeds – another marvellous way to obtain the omega-3 fatty acids (also contains omega-6 and omega-9) is to grind up ¼ cup (recommended therapeutic daily dose) of flaxseeds in a small coffee grinder and add to smoothies. Flax contains lignans, which are plant estrogen, antioxidants that are known for their prostate and breast cancer prevention properties. Additionally, flaxseeds contain protein, B vitamins, potassium, lecithin, magnesium and zinc. Good for reducing the pain and inflammation of arthritis, found to lower cholesterol and triglyceride levels, as well as maintaining bowels. Great to grind up and put in a morning smoothie (see smoothie recipe).

Garlic – one of garlic's greatest values is its natural antibiotic effect. Did you know it was used to prevent gangrene during World War I? Garlic is very effective with fungal infections like candida,

common athlete's foot and vaginitis. Research is being done using garlic to destroy certain viruses like herpes, fever blisters and smallpox, as well as colds and flu. Another great way to build up the immune system.

Hemp seeds – hemp seeds are a must for vegans as they are an incredible source of biologically available and easy-to-digest protein containing all 10 essential amino acids. Just 3 tablespoons of hemp seeds contain 11 grams of protein. The 3:1 ratio of omega-6 to omega-3 fat in the seeds enables a healthy anti-inflammatory potential affect largely due to an especially beneficial type of omega-6 fat known as GLA (gamma linolenic acid), which is not typically found in foods.

GLA benefits:

GLA supports a healthy metabolism and facilitates fat burning (some people who struggle with weight loss despite eating a healthy diet get a weight loss boost simply by adding GLA to their diets.)

◆ GLA has been noted to help relieve PMS

◆ GLA supports healthy hair, nails and skin

◆ GLA decreases the tendency of inflammation in general. This can be helpful to anyone with an inflammatory condition such as asthma, MS, fibromyalgia, arthritis, etc.

◆ GLA helps lower bad LDL cholesterol and improve cholesterol ratio

NOTE: GLA can also be obtained from supplements such as Borage Seed Oil and Evening Primrose Oil, found in Udo's Oil.

Additionally, hemp seeds are rich in vitamin E and an array of minerals including zinc, calcium, phosphorous, magnesium and iron.

Krill Oil – if you are not opposed to a high-quality animal-based omega-3 supplement, krill is your best option. Rich in essential EPA and DHA in a double-chain phospholipid structure, making it a superior choice over the other omega-3 fish oils. Another important factor is krill oil contains vitamins E, A, D and natural astaxanthin, which is a powerful antioxidant and helps protect the oil from going rancid. Research using the ORAC (Oxygen Radical Absorbency Capacity) scale finds krill oil 48 times more potent than fish oil.[18]

Omega-3 fatty acids are necessary for human health and development but the body cannot make them. Instead we have to make sure our diets contain foods rich in these fatty acids or by supplementation. Supplementing with omega-3 from krill oil, which has these fatty acids in "phospholipid" form rather than the lesser "triglyceride" form found in fish oils, allows the body to absorb them more efficiently and easily.

There are several key health benefits from supplementing with krill oil:[19]

◆ **Heart:** higher levels of HDL ("good") cholesterol reduces the risk of heart disease and a recent study[1] has shown that supplementation with krill oil can increase this "good" cholesterol by 14% compared with just 3% using fish oils.

Furthermore, a reduction in triglycerides in the blood is also known to reduce the risks of heart disease and the study showed that supplementing with krill oil reduced triglycerides by 13% as opposed to 1% using fish oil.

◆ **Brain:** the fatty acid DHA is an important building block in the brain and is the most important essential nutrient in a young infant's diet. As DHA from krill oil absorbs better into the body, this is a superior source of fatty acids for brain development.

◆ **Vision:** krill oil supplies easily absorbed EPA and DHA as well as a powerful anti-oxidant known as Astaxanthin. DHA is known for its support of vision and can help in reducing sight degeneration. Astaxanthin provides an anti-oxidant shield against retinal damage from UV light.

◆ **Joints:** the omega-3 in krill oil supports the body's anti-inflammatory responses and can help to reduce joint pain, speed recovery and keep joints supple. In a comparison of scientific studies into the effects of fish oils and krill oil on joint pain, krill oil outperforms fish oils and at a lower dose.

Lemons – a wonderful cleansing and alkalinizing food. Using the lemon peel gives you 5–10 times more vitamins than just the juice alone.

TIP: To add the value of lemon peels into your diet, simply wash the outer skin and place lemon in your freezer. Once the lemon is frozen use your grater and shred the whole lemon. Sprinkle the grated lemon in and on your food. Great in salads, ice cream, soup, smoothies, rice, fish dishes, even whisky!

The grated lemon will perk up most food with a fresh unexpected taste. I like to freeze lemons before I travel and throw them in with the foods I am carrying on board to keep things nice and cold. Then once I arrive at my destination the lemons have thawed, and I have them ready for lemon water the next morning no matter where in the world I have landed!

Lemon water is an integral part of doing PURE 5:2. Begin each day adding the juice of one lemon to 16–32 oz. of warm water and drink first thing in the morning. This will help to move bowels, cleanse kidneys and urinary tract, alkalize the body, kick-start the liver, remove mucus, and hydrate the body.

Also, make up a pitcher of water and stir in the juice of 4–6 lemons and drink throughout your day, especially on a "2-day." Lemon juice acts like a cleanser. According to Jethro Kloss, author of *Back to Eden*, lemons prevent bacteria buildup and help to rid the body of impurities. Lemon water is a great way to alkalinize as well as being high in potassium. Use lemon water as a tonic for indigestion, heartburn, bloating, gas, and cramps. We like to add Manuka honey for additional benefits. To preserve the enzymes, don't heat water past 118/48° and never use ice.

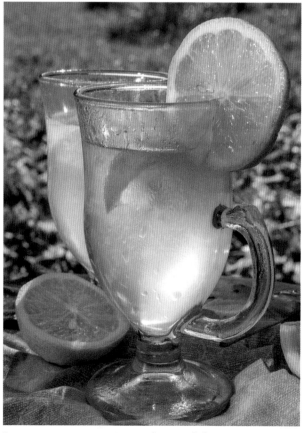

Lemon water — an integral part of doing PURE 5:2

Manuka honey, unique to New Zealand, has incredible and reliable health-giving properties and can be used as a natural remedy to assist with a variety of health conditions. Manuka honey has been known to be effective combating bacteria responsible for sore throats and wound infections. This honey has also proven to be effective in helping the natural healing of skin ulcers, burns, boils, cracked skin and even the "superbug" MRSA. For only four weeks during midsummer, the manuka bush is covered in white flowers. During this time bees work tirelessly gathering the honey from the manuka flower. Methylglyoxal forms naturally in the manuka nectar, ready for collection by the bees.

Probiotics – it is essential to take probiotics when one takes any kind of antibiotic to help maintain the "friendly bacteria" in the digestive tract. Just taking yogurt or kefir isn't strong enough. Probiotics help to promote the proper digestion of food and is a great aid when undigested food causes the body to produce histamine, resulting in allergic symptoms. Probiotics are great for all kinds of stomach upsets, and especially good to take when stomach flu is going around or at the first hints of food poisoning (see fermented foods).

Probiotics are great for all kinds of stomach upsets, and especially good to take when stomach flu is going around

Shiitake mushrooms – a great superfood, containing eighteen amino acids, B vitamins, and a polysaccharide known as lentinan, which increases T-cell function strengthening the immune system. Shiitakes are also known to be very effective in treating cancer.

Spirulina – according to David Sandoval, author of *The Green Food Bible,* this is nature's richest source of plant protein, containing more than three times the protein in fish, poultry or red meat. Spirulina is also very high in calcium (containing five times more calcium than whole milk), beta-carotene and essential fatty acids.

Spirulina is commonly used for its antioxidant protection, as a weight loss aid, protein powder, energy supplement and immune system enhancer. Spirulina is a whole food, so you can safely eat as much or little as you like with or without meals. Spirulina is a key ingredient in our daily smoothie.

Truly one of my all time favorite superfoods; I gained tremendous benefit using spirulina when I was recovering from being poisoned, as well as

helping me to heal from extreme hypoglycemia. It is an immune system builder, a blood purifier and detoxifier. Spirulina is an excellent way to get a range of minerals. Finding whole food sources of minerals can be challenging with our depleted soils. Since this is an algae grown in water, we bypass the depleted soil issue. Seaweeds in general are loaded with minerals. Mineral deficiencies account for all kinds of hidden health issues. Spirulina is an excellent source of pure organic, easy-to-digest minerals that the body utilizes well. Be sure to pick a source that is not coming from radiation contaminated waters (since Fukushima).

NOTE: To order our favorite PURE spirulina, see Chapter 6, *Get Equipped.*

Fresh turmeric is loaded with powerful antioxidant abilities thanks to its yellow-colored active ingredient, known as curcumin. Aside from being a great antioxidant, this profound root (in the ginger family) has anti-inflammatory, antibacterial, stomach soothing, and liver and heart protecting effects. Used to ease joint pain and inflammation experienced with arthritis. Another promising aspect of this spectacular natural wonder is to reduce the ability of the blood to form clots, helping to improve circulation and offer potential protection against heart attacks and strokes. Known to have anti-cancer activity, much research is going into to discovering more about turmeric's role in disease prevention.

CAUTION: People with the following conditions should avoid turmeric: those with congestive heart disease with an unknown cause, and people with painful gallstones, obstructive jaundice, acute bilious colic, or toxic liver disorders.

Udo's Choice Ultimate Oil Blend – The ultimate source of omega-3, -6, and -9, and especially popular for raw foodies, vegans and vegetarians. It is the UK's market leading nutritional oil blend and recommended by one of the UK's most recognized nutritionists, Patrick Holford, in his new book, *The Holford Diet.* Udo's Choice delivers a balanced 2:1:1 ratio of the Essential Fatty Acids (EFAs) omega-3 and -6, and the beneficial fatty acid omega-9. It is a unique blend of certified organic flax, sunflower, coconut and sesame oils, with unrefined oils from the germs of rice and oats, evening primrose oil and non-GM lecithin.

Walnuts – this has now become our all-time favorite nut. It's no accident walnuts are shaped to look like the brain. Maybe that was by design to remind us to eat lots of them for brain health. Recent studies show that walnuts may even help fight major depression. The omega-3's make it easier for brain cell receptors to process mood-related signals from neighboring neurons. Other benefits include potential for: lowering cholesterol; protection from heart disease, stroke and some cancers; reduction of inflammatory diseases such as arthritis; plus it has been found to reverse brain aging in rats. The research on the rats found that more was not better when it comes to walnuts. One ounce, or 7–9 walnuts, a day is the recommended amount to keep the oils in the right balance. When you think of food as medicine, and walnuts are certainly medicinal in their effect, you don't want to overdose! A little bit goes a long way. We suggest adding some walnuts in your morning smoothie or into salad dressings.

> *It's no accident walnuts are shaped to look like the brain. Maybe that was by design, to remind us to eat an ounce (7–9 walnuts) a day for brain health.*

Wheatgrass – a potent detoxifier rich with chlorophyll and a wide variety of vitamins and minerals much like barley grass. Served "fresh" at juice bars for over 30 years as one of nature's most rejuvenating foods. When fresh is not available, powdered Kamut is. Very convenient if you don't have a juicer or when you travel.

NOTE: see Chapter 6, *Get Equipped* for ordering information.

Getting Enough Calcium and Protein

The milk industry would lead us to believe that animal dairy milk is the only way to get adequate supplies of calcium. However, rest assured that there are many foods that supply the nutritional components found in dairy milk. Almonds, beans, peas, coconuts, spirulina, whole grains and greens such as kale supply ample amounts of calcium. There have been many studies done proving that without the heavy intake of animal protein (that actually robs the body of calcium to be able to digest these foods), we don't require as much calcium as was once believed.

In terms of protein, the time the body requires the most amount of protein due to the rapid growth period is in infancy. It takes a human baby 180 days to double its birth weight. However,

did you know that 1 cup of human breast milk only contains 2.4 gm. of protein and 80 mg of calcium? Think about that! The human baby with blossoming growth, rapid weight gain and developing organs only requires 2.4 grams of protein per cup! Only 5% of the calories come from protein. (Almond milk contains only 2 grams of protein per cup, coming in very close to human milk protein content.)

Cows, on the other hand, produce milk with 8.5 gm. of protein and 288 mg of calcium. That is a big difference — roughly four times the amount of protein and more than three times the amount of calcium. A baby calf doubles its birth weight in only 47 days, which is approximately four times as fast as us humans. Because of this rapid development, the protein in milk for baby calves contains 15% protein, as compared to 5% for baby humans. Guess where the mama cow gets the protein to produce the protein found in her milk. You guessed it, from eating green grass! That's right. That big old heifer cow gets all the protein she requires to make all that meat and bones from grass! So where on earth did we get the notion that human beings needed to wean off of mother's milk onto an ongoing diet including the milk from the mother of a baby calf?! Just what is the wisdom of that?

Dr. McDougall points out he does not see diseases of deficiency in his patients. Rather, he sees diseases of excess. Therefore, he concludes that feeding an overly concentrated food such as cow's milk to people (infants, children, and adults) promotes diseases of excess. Studies show a concern about diabetes (there is about 2 ½ tsp. of sugar in 8 oz. of milk) and leukemia in children possibly being linked to excess dairy consumption. Dairy is one of the most prevalent foods causing allergic reactions resulting in symptoms such as ear, nose and throat infections.

Foods rich with calcium include: almonds, barley grass, blackstrap molasses, broccoli, butternut squash, coconut milk, collards, dried figs, kale, kamut-wheatgrass, oranges, navy beans, spirulina, sunflower seeds, and tahini.

Foods for Preventing and Impacting Cancer

Approximately 35% of cancers are related to nutritional factors. Here is a list of foods rich in nutrients to help protect the body on a cellular level from free radical damage.

1. **Almonds** and almond butter for the vitamin E

2. **Berries**, especially blueberries and cranberries. Berries contain nutrients that help to prevent carcinogens from binding to the DNA in cells. When it comes to berries, blueberries are the pick of the crop because of their high antioxidant content. Also consider using (organic only) raspberries, strawberries and goji berries. When in season, include them into your daily diet. Did you know that strawberries are one of the most heavily sprayed of all crops?

3. **Cruciferous vegetables** contain extremely beneficial phytonutrients that inhibit the effects of carcinogens as well as stimulating the body's detoxification enzymes. Optimally it is wise to choose three or four servings per week of arugula, bok choy, broccoli, Brussels sprouts, cabbage, cauliflower, collard greens, kale, neeps, parsnips, radishes, rutabaga, swede, turnips, watercress.

4. **Flax seeds** – especially good for breast cancer prevention because of the lignans and omega-3 oils inhibiting cancer cell proliferation. They also reduce inflammation, thus decreasing the possibility of cellular mutations. One quarter of a cup of ground flax seeds per day is considered a therapeutic dose.

5. **Grapefruits** are high in Vitamin C, preventing cancers of the stomach, colon, esophagus, bladder and cervix. Citrus fruits are valuable for their limonoids, known to inhibit activation of cancer cells. Aim to include grapefruits, lemons, limes, oranges, and tangerines into your daily diet.

6. **Green tea** contains compounds known as catechins, thought to inhibit cancer cell growth and mutations. Found to be helpful for breast, colon, ovarian, prostate and lung cancer prevention. The flavonoids found in tea are known for neutralizing destructive free radicals. Some suggest drinking two cups a day of green, black, or oolong teas. However, my favorite tea is Rooibos because it is naturally caffeine free, contains no oxalic acid and is very low in tannin. Rooibos tea is very high in anti-oxidants. In my opinion it tastes much better than other black or green teas and is overall better for you. You can find Rooibos in health food stores.

7. **Pomegranates** contain ellagic acid which is a powerhouse phytonutrient shown in scientific studies to inhibit cancer cell growth and deactivate cancer-causing compounds. Use pomegranate seeds in smoothies, on top of yogurt or in salads. Other foods containing ellagic acid are raspberries, blackberries, strawberries, walnuts, pecans, cranberries, and grapes.

8. **Sweet potatoes and green leafy vegetables** for beta-carotene, especially good for breast cancer prevention.

9. **Tomatoes** have received lots of press because they contain lycopene, a wonderful cell membrane protector. Cooking tomatoes breaks down the cell walls and releases more lycopenes. Lycopenes have been found to be helpful for (among other things) prostate cancer (cooked tomatoes four times a week provides a beneficial amount).

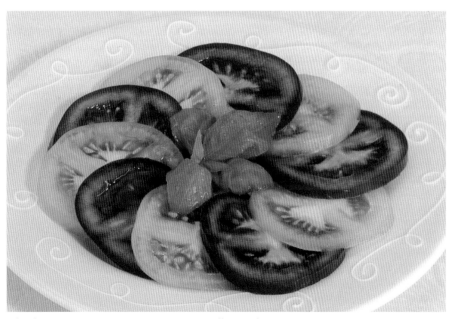

The lycopene in tomatoes protects cell membranes.

10. **Turmeric** contains curcumin, an active ingredient curtailing inflammations, and high in antioxidants, shown to help prevent breast, colon, stomach, liver and lung cancers.

11. **Salmon (wild only)** – low Vitamin D levels have been linked to breast and colon cancers, and wild salmon is a good source. Few foods contain Vitamin D, so supplementing is needed.

12. **Sprouts** are a nutrient-dense, enzyme-rich, and phytochemically powerful food. Did you know that certain varieties of sprouts yield 10 to 30 times more nutritional value than the best organic vegetables you can grow in the best organic soil in your yard? In 1992, John Hopkins research found a diet high in cruciferous vegetables, especially broccoli, as having some of the most potent anti-cancer activity. Additionally, further research uncovered that sprouted broccoli seeds have over ten times the phytochemical ability to kill cancer.

Surprisingly, sunflsower seed and pea sprouts contain approximately 30 times more nutritional value than organic vegetables. Sprouting is one of the best ways to get high nutrient dense food into your diet. Eating sprouts daily can provide:

♦ Support for cell regeneration

♦ Powerful sources of antioxidants, minerals, vitamins and enzymes that protect against free radical damage

♦ Alkalinizing effect on your body, helping to protect against disease, especially cancer (as many tumors are thought to grow in an acid environment)

♦ A rich source of oxygen, known to protect against abnormal cell growth, viruses and bacteria that cannot survive in an oxygen-rich environment

It is possible to sprout a wide variety of different beans, nuts, seeds and grains. Sprouting is inexpensive, simple to do, and can be grown inside. This is especially important for those in darker, colder climates and those worldwide who suffer from malnutrition and hunger due to poverty.

A Great Way to Preserve Fresh Juice

This is a great idea I read in a little book called *Living Food Lifestyle* by Elizabeth Miller. If you like to drink plenty of fresh juice throughout the day but only have time to juice in the morning, purchase a stainless steel-lined thermos. Rinse it out, leaving a few drops of water inside, and lay it horizontally in the freezer overnight. The frozen drops will help preserve your juice. Fill it all the way to the top the next morning with your fresh juice. Place the lid on tightly, making a seal, as the juice will actually overflow as you screw the

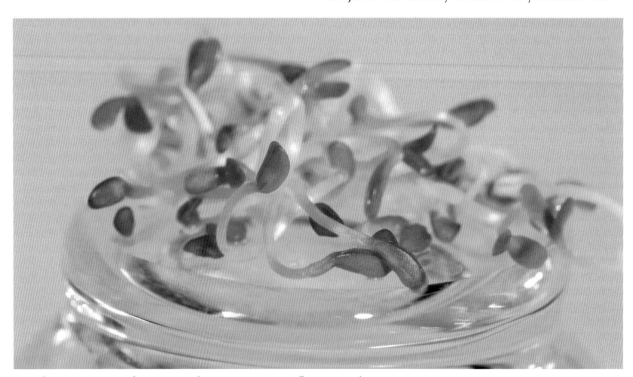

Our favorite sprouts, for taste and nutrients, are sunflower seed sprouts.

lid on. This will, in a sense, vacuum-pack the juice and preserve it (up to 10 hours) so you can enjoy it all day. Seal it quickly after each drink, as oxygen is what destroys the nutrition in the juice.

If your juicer is not designed to juice wheatgrass, try wrapping the wheatgrass blades inside a piece of lettuce. Roll it up like a burrito and stuff it down the chute of your juicer. Some folks say this works better than buying a new juicer!

Quick Tip on Soaking and Sprouting

It is important to soak nuts and seeds to wash off naturally occurring growth inhibitors. These inhibitors prevent them from sprouting prematurely, should drops of water penetrate the skins. Additionally, soaking and sprouting helps to pre-digest food, as the fats are broken down into fatty acids and the proteins into amino acids.

Most small nuts and legumes like sunflower seeds, lentils, mung and adzuki only require two to three hours of soaking. Over soaking causes waterlogging and they do not sprout well. It is best to soak almonds up to 24 hours (rinsing twice a day).

Cover nuts, seeds, and legumes with water and soak for desired time. Pour through wire mesh strainer and rinse well. Let the sprouting "living food" keep bursting forth right in the mesh strainer by sitting it inside a stainless steel bowl. Rinse twice a day by filling the bowl with enough water to give what you are sprouting a little bath! Let them bathe only long enough for you to stir them up. Drain and put them back out to sunbathe, sitting back inside the strainer.

NOTE: Our favorite sprouts, for taste and nutrients, are sunflower seed sprouts.

About Proper Food Combining

The issue about food combining really has to do with enzymes. The body uses different enzymes to digest different types of food. Eating the wrong combinations can cause foods to be retained longer in the stomach, causing them to rot and ferment and in some cases lead to a condition called leaky gut syndrome. Not a pretty picture!

Ideally, it is best to eat fruit alone, especially melons. Remember this one: "Eat melons alone or leave them alone." If you violate this rule, watch out, you could be in for some serious indigestion and gas.

Keep it simple:

Grains, nuts, seeds and legumes combine well with all veggies. All veggies do well together.

Watch for bloating and gas as signs of poor combinations, assimilation, and digestion. Headaches, tummy aches, gas pains and spaciness are all signs that can point to the fallout of poor combinations, food sensitivities or allergies. Of course, these symptoms can also indicate other issues.

The Hazards of Using a Microwave

In a nutshell, the use of microwaves changes the molecular structure of foods. Dr. Lita Lee, in her book, *Health Effects of Microwave Radiation— Microwave Ovens*, stated that every microwave oven leaks electromagnetic radiation. She feels that every substance cooked in a microwave converts it to a "dangerous organ-toxic and carcinogenic product."

One has to wonder why the Soviet Union banned the use of microwaves in 1976. I suggest you go to **mercola.com/article/microwave/hazards.htm** and read this very informative article, which will technically explain how a microwave works and renders food harmful.

Based on conclusions from Swiss, Russian and German scientific clinical studies, we can no longer ignore the issues posed by household microwave ovens.

10 Reasons to Throw Out Your Microwave Oven (Copied with permission from: **healthfree.com/paa/paa0001.htm**)

1. Continually eating food processed from a microwave oven causes long-term permanent brain damage by "shorting out" electrical impulses in the brain (de-polarizing or de-magnetizing the brain tissue).

2. The human body cannot metabolize (break down) the unknown by-products created in microwaved food.

3. Male and female hormone production is shut down and/or altered by continually eating microwaved foods.

4. The effects of microwaved food by-products are residual (long term, permanent) within the human body.

5. Minerals, vitamins, and nutrients of all microwaved foods are reduced or altered

so that the human body gets little or no benefit, or the human body absorbs altered compounds that cannot be broken down.

6. The minerals in vegetables are altered into cancerous free radicals when cooked in microwave ovens.

7. Microwaved foods cause stomach and intestinal cancerous growths (tumors). This may explain the rapidly increasing rate of colon cancer in America.

8. The prolonged eating of microwaved foods causes cancerous cells to increase in human blood.

9. Continual ingestion of microwaved food causes immune system deficiencies through lymph gland and blood serum alterations.

10. Eating microwaved food causes loss of memory, concentration, emotional instability and decrease of intelligence.

Have you tossed out your microwave oven yet?

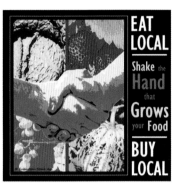

Words to live by; artwork by Rebecca Simpson of suburbanstoneage.com

What About Eating at Restaurants?

In the rapid pace of our culture, eating at restaurants is a fact of life. However, did you stop and think about another fact concerning restaurant eating? Most restaurants use microwaves to prepare some portion of the meals they serve. Most sauces and salad dressings (when they aren't made from scratch) contain hidden MSG. The more delicious the food tastes, the more you can bet food additives, colorings, preservatives, GMO foods, highly processed salt and oils, lots of sugar, etc. are sure to be found. So what to do? Relax and simply make the best choices you can.

If you would prefer not to eat unhealthy oils, you can carry your own salad dressing in a small glass jar or just use fresh lemons to squeeze on salads. You can bring your own water in a stainless steel thermos, when possible. Ask if the food you are interested in is microwaved. Eat simply, but most of all try to enjoy your time out. Also bring some nuts to eat so when they bring the bread to the table and

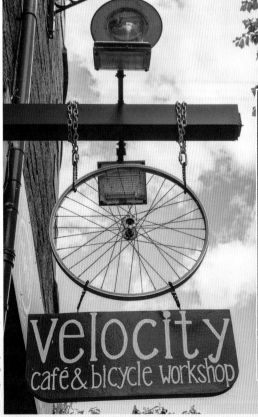

Velocity sign photo by Robyn Randolph

Velocity Cafe in Inverness uses PURE organic food from Maggie's Farm.

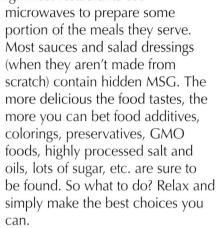

Chef Wendy uses Maggie's fresh-farmed produce at her B-and-B restaurant, Rockvilla, in Locharron.

32

others dive in you can have an option. Or eat a handful of nuts before entering the restaurant so you won't be tempted to overeat or eat high-glycemic carbs.

My biggest vice in life used to be eating at restaurants. Before I became well-educated about processed food, nutrition and healthy choices, I ate out at least twice a week without a care in the world; bite after bite, oblivious to what I was ingesting, like millions of people every day. Now I find the power of information has transformed my eating habits on many levels, especially at restaurants. I find that as my palate has changed, so has my choice in restaurants. In this natural evolution, I find I'm naturally attracted to ordering differently. As my own cooking has evolved, I find that when I do eat out, foods taste too salty or too sweet, or too oily, or too heavy. The desire to go out is less and less. It all gets much simpler over time.

If there was just one thing I wish EVERY restaurant would do, it would be to switch over to Himalayan or Celtic Sea salt. When possible ask restaurant owners to consider making that switch. Just like we now see gluten-free listed on menus, let's encourage restaurant owners to make a note on their menus when they state they serve only the finest ingredients that they can also say: "including Himalayan salt!"

Whenever possible pick a restaurant that uses local, organic PURE foods. You cast your vote every time you choose how and where to spend your money. Will it be to nourish you and your local farmers and community?

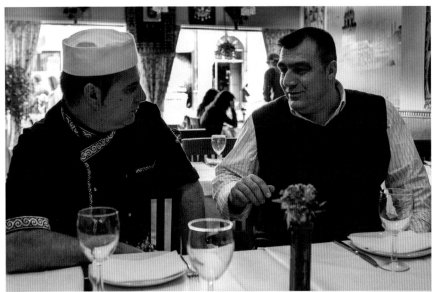

Aspendos in Inverness uses local PURE foods to create amazing intuitive Turkish cuisine.

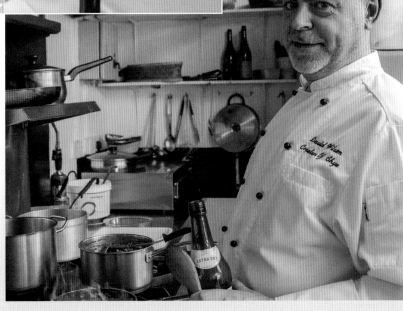

Creelers, on Skye, uses fresh local fish and produce to create intuitively healthy dishes. We use chef David's delicious Cajun spice mix in our dehydrated crackers.

Support Your Local Organic Farmers and the Restaurants Using Their Food

Here are pictures of a few of our wonderful Scottish Highlands farmers who grow the organic foods that go to the local chefs, so they can prepare fresh, PURE foods at the restaurants we choose to support, here in the Highlands.

These photos came from two weeks of interviews we did throughout the Highlands of Northern Scotland. We loved meeting several of the local organic farmers and learning tips and tasting samples of their nourishing foods. We also went to some of the local restaurants the farmers supply and watched the chefs use their highly refined and intuitive cooking skills to create delicious, life-enhancing cuisine.

Peter and Therese Muskus of Laikenbuie Organic Farm in Nairn.

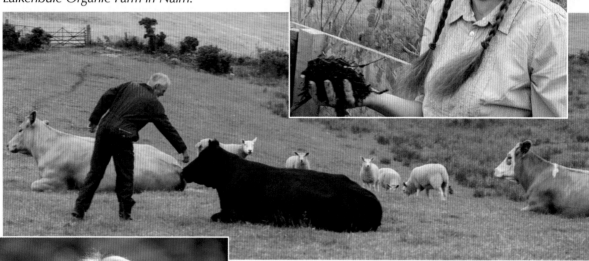

Maggie of Clachandreggy Farms in Inverness, growing macro sprouts for local restaurants.

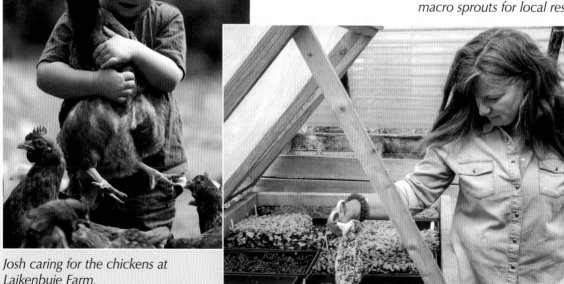

Josh caring for the chickens at Laikenbuie Farm.

34

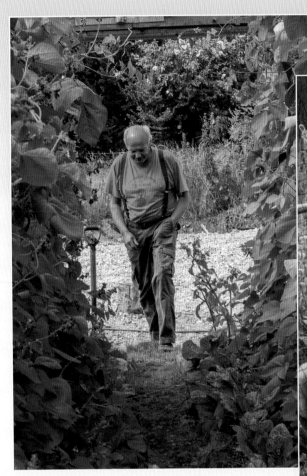

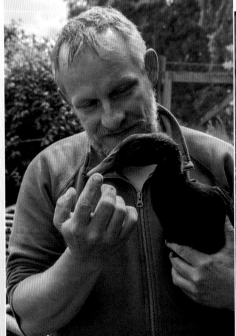

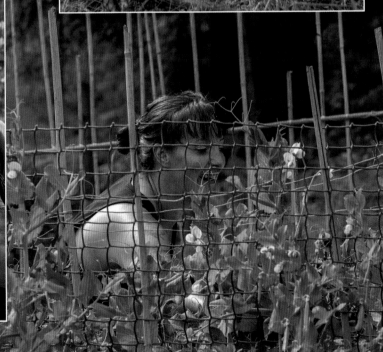

Christopher Raymont of Newbold House.
He was the head gardener
of Findhorn for 13 years.

Donnie Mcleod of Mcleod Organics
in Ardersier.

Ludwig Appeltan uses ducks
for natural pest control in his
permaculture gardens in Forres.

Jacqui McKinnon of Strathconon Organix Farm (in Strathconon).

About Salt

It has become apparent that table salt as we have known it is not on the must-get list. We all know that packaged foods contain plenty of it, and there is the heavy-handed use of it at restaurants. One thing many folks don't realize is that when the words "sea salt" are used on supposed health food packages, it doesn't mean that this salt is any better. This salt usually has gone through a process of being mechanically harvested from dirt or concrete basins. Then it is put through several artificial processes and heated to the point of altering its molecular structure. This robs the salt of its essential minerals. The salt is further assaulted when chemical additives are used to make it free flowing, bleached to make it pure white, and iodized!

Himalayan Pink Crystal Salt is my favorite choice, having a wonderful subtle crunchy texture, raw or cooked, and is rich in minerals including calcium, magnesium, potassium, copper and iron. Formed millions of years ago and harvested from the foothills of the Himalayas, this salt is unrefined and truly an earthly treasure.

If we could just get every restaurant owner to switch to healthy salt, what a difference it would make. Encourage your local restaurants to upgrade and to note the healthy change on their menus.

Potential health benefits of using natural Himalayan Crystal Salt may include:

◆ Maintaining proper water levels within the body
◆ Encouraging stable pH balance in the cells and brain
◆ Contributing to balanced blood sugar
◆ Anti-aging
◆ Aiding with increased nutrient absorption in the intestinal tract
◆ Supporting vascular health
◆ Boosting respiratory function
◆ Decreasing sinus issues
◆ Reducing muscle cramps
◆ Increasing bone strength
◆ Naturally promoting healthy sleep patterns
◆ Creating a healthy libido

One of the best forms of naturally-occurring salt in the correct mineral balance can be found in celery. It is wise to drink celery juice often and add it to other vegetable juices.

What About Wheat and Going Against the Grain?

If you told me I had to pick only one food (well maybe two) for the rest of my life, I would undoubtedly say: homemade bread fresh out of the oven with butter! That is, if health didn't matter and I was just going for taste and comfort alone!

People today act as if bread is one of the four main food groups! Well it isn't, and honestly shouldn't be considered on the charts at all. Not after you learn what I am about to tell you…and let me say ahead: "sorry to say, but…"

The cross breeding of wheat began in the 50s when scientists were looking for ways to improve wheat growing. They didn't realize then that this cross breeding would introduce compounds that would wreak such havoc on the human digestive system.

As cardiologist Dr. William Davis noted in his book, *Wheat Belly: Lose the Wheat, Lose the Weight and Find Your Path Back to Health*, today's hybridized wheat has been mutated with a toxin known as sodium azide. It also goes through a gamma irradiation process during manufacturing. He points out that today's hybridized wheat contains proteins in forms that are too difficult for us to digest, thus we are seeing the resulting rise in "gluten sensitivity".

Gluten is a protein comprised of gliadin and glutenin. It is also found in rye, barley, and spelt. Gluten helps dough to rise and gives it shape and texture. Alessio Fasano, the Medical Director for The University of Maryland's Center for Celiac Research, says that no one can properly digest gluten because we don't have the enzymes to properly break it down. This then, sets off an immunogenic response triggering systemic inflammation, leading to a range of autoimmune diseases such as celiac, rheumatoid arthritis, and irritable bowel syndrome.

Gliadin has been accused of creating leaky gut syndrome as well as creating a morphine-like compound after eating, resulting in an addictive type of effect. Recent studies reveal the alarming rise of gluten sensitivity in one form or another. Gluten-free products and actual sections in grocery stores are now becoming commonplace.

Wheat is at the top of the list for raising blood sugar and is getting kicked off the grocery list of all those with blood sugar issues. As more and more people are being diagnosed with high cholesterol and pre-diabetes, wheat is being examined for the role it plays as a major contributing factor. Just two slices of wheat bread can trigger increased blood sugar levels higher than one candy bar! Who knew? Don't be fooled, whole wheat bread is no better than the lesser of two evils.

Dr. William Davis' mantra is lose wheat, lose weight. We would have to agree and to that we would add: "and gain health"! Our new mantra: *"Lose wheat, lose weight, gain health"*!

10 Signs of Gluten Intolerance

According to Dr. Amy Myers, if you have any of the following symptoms, it could be a sign that you have gluten intolerance:

1. Digestive issues including gas, bloating, diarrhea or constipation (commonly seen in children) after eating gluten.

2. Keratosis pilaris, also known as "chicken skin," commonly found on the back of arms. Gluten damages the gut, creating fat malabsorption, which leads to fatty acid and vitamin A deficiency, resulting in bumpy skin on the back of the arms.

3. Fatigue, brain fog, or feeling tired after eating a meal that contains gluten.

4. Diagnosis of an autoimmune disease such as Hashimoto's thyroiditis, rheumatoid arthritis, ulcerative colitis, lupus, psoriasis, scleroderma or multiple sclerosis.

5. Neurologic symptoms such as dizziness, or a feeling of being off-balance.

6. Hormone imbalances such as PMS, PCOS, or unexplained infertility.

7. Migraine headaches.

8. Diagnosis of chronic fatigue or fibromyalgia, which can be a mis-diagnosis by a doctor who cannot pinpoint the cause of your fatigue or pain.

9. Inflammation, swelling, or pain in joints such as fingers, knees or hips.

10. Anxiety, depression, mood swings, and ADD.

R Is for RAW and E Is for Enzyme-rich

Raw, raw, raw! Why eat raw?

If the food we eat is irradiated (treating food with specific ionizing radiation to prolong shelf life and destroy microorganisms, halting spoilage by retarding enzyme action) microwaved, processed, artificial, chemically thriving, over-salted, overcooked, oily food, then guess what? We are eating dead food, devoid of any enzymes. All food, no matter if it is PURE and organic, that is cooked past 48C/118F destroys all enzymes, and enzymes are what feed and nourish every cell in our bodies.

What is all this talk about enzymes? Is this yet another food fad? Enzymes are what eating raw is all about. Enzymes are foundational for proper body functioning. Put simply, no enzymes, no life; the more enzymes, the more life. Enzymes are found in every cell of anything that lives. They are composed of amino acids, which are the structural units of all proteins. Enzymes are catalysts in the metabolic process. They jump-start chemical reactions responsible for building up new tissue growth as well as breaking down substances, as in digestion.

Enzymes have a wide range of applications in body processes; therefore we contain over three thousand kinds of enzymes, with each enzyme performing a different job. They are like construction workers busy building and repairing parts of our bodies. Enzymes are critical to our well-being so that when the quantities decrease, there is a noticeable decrease in health as well. Injury, illness, stress and aging all play a role in decreasing the amount and potency of enzymes.

Because enzymes are very sensitive to heat, it is critical to eat food in a non-heated, thus non-deadened state. Live, raw foods, such as sprouts, provide the best source of enzymes. Next best would be raw organic juices. To experience more vitality, energy and aliveness in your body, simply decrease cooked and dead food and replace with raw food.

The first function of enzymes is to help break down our ingested food. But what if the food you just ingested was cooked food? Then you are asking your body to provide existing enzymes for this purpose, which causes a deficit from your body's cells.

There are specific enzymes to help break down specific foods. For example, certain enzymes known as protease help break down proteins into amino acids and others known as lipase break down fats into fatty acids.

When you ingest a raw food, it comes intact with the proper enzymes to break that food down. It is how that food was designed in nature. When you eat a man-made food, full of chemicals, over-processed or cooked, it is void of the enzymes to break that food down. Instead your body will kick up random enzymes from your reserve of enzymes that are not fully capable of breaking down that food.

As we grow older, the body begins to produce considerably fewer enzymes due to the aging process. This is why we see elderly people having more of a challenge digesting and processing their food as each year passes. As long as people keep eating dead food they can expect to have the related problems that go with enzyme depletion. Remember then, that adding enzyme-rich foods to your diet helps to prevent robbing your body of these vital life-giving elements. Eating raw food means it comes already intact with the proper enzymes to help break that food down.

Asking your body to supply the enzymes creates an unnecessary task that is wearing over time. This can result in a lack of energy, digestive ailments, chronic illness and disease. The first thing I hear people say once they have been on a mostly raw diet for as little as one week is: "I can't believe how much more energy I have!" Cooked food creates more waste by-products and toxins that the body has to work harder to try to eliminate. If optimum health is what you are after, then eating a diet rich in raw foods will take you to a wholesome new level.[20–24]

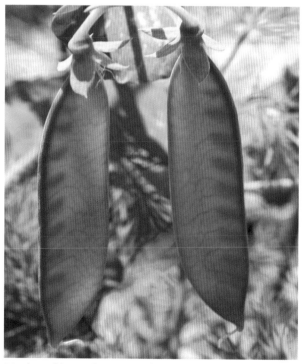

Nothing like picking your food fresh off the vine!

Aging, Enzymes and a Case for Raw Cuisine!

What exactly is old age and how do we do that aging thing gracefully? Let's face the fact, we aren't getting chronologically any younger and all the face creams in the world are not going to prevent the wrinkles of time. However, studies show that despite the progressive impairment of mitochondrial function, increased oxidative stress, and immune activation that characterizes old age...we have the power to influence these things by modification of our nutritional intake.

You have come a long way, baby, and now it is up to you to do what you can do. Not what a pill, cream or an advertisement leads you to hope you can do. Hoping and wanting, means doing, in order to have or be. Think about that. Until your mitochondria show you otherwise, you are the one lifting the fork to your face! In others words, in the here and now, only you can do what it takes to feed yourself well.

Animal studies show caloric restriction reduces oxidative stress, leading to longer life expectancy. Whether the majority of people can live with caloric restriction or not may never be proven, given the addiction people have to carbohydrates. Perhaps psychologically it is easier to accept the idea of upgrading to better quality foods as opposed to the concept of caloric restriction primarily from carbohydrates. That is where learning about AGE (advanced glycation end products) comes in.

Advanced glycation end products (AGEs) are a group of macromolecules that are formed by the non-enzymatic glycation of proteins, lipids, and nucleic acids (what happens when protein or lipid molecules bond with sugar molecules without the controlling action of an enzyme). There are two main sources of AGEs we are exposed to: exogenous AGEs ingested in foods and endogenous AGEs formed in the body. Search no further than the Western diet to find an abundance of exogenous AGEs.

AGEs develop when food is processed at elevated temperatures. Methods such as deep-frying, broiling, roasting, grilling, barbecuing, as well as making pasteurized dairy products, cheeses, sausages, processed meats, and commercial breakfast cereals, all form AGEs. AGEs increase oxidative stress. They therefore can accelerate multisystem decline that occurs with aging. This suggests not only reducing the intake of known AGEs but increasing high-enzymatic raw foods to promote healthy aging and greater longevity, as well.

Radiation Protection in the Age of Fukushima

"There is no safe amount of radiation. Even small amounts do harm."

— *Dr. Linus Pauling*

"Nuclear power is one hell of a way to boil water."

— *Albert Einstein*

Living on planet Earth, it is impossible to escape radiation. We are continually subject to background radiation from cosmic rays and the radiation from natural radioactive decay of minerals on earth. Additionally, dangerous man-made sources of radiation now contaminate our environment. Since July 1945 there have been over 2000 atomic bombs exploded on Earth. The 541 above-ground nuclear bombs tested in the 1950s and 60s released huge amounts of finely powdered radioactive debris. Concurrent with this development was the creation of an entire nuclear industry, consisting of mining and refining and transmutation of radioactive fuels, construction of over 500 nuclear reactors and building of tens of thousands of nuclear warheads. To top it off, even so-called "conventional weapons" now utilize radioactive "depleted" uranium. This is turned into a powdery toxic dust when used and has widely contaminated countries like Iraq.

Just as we have polluted our planet with chemical pollution from factories, automobiles, industrial agriculture, etc., we have also contaminated the Earth with man-made sources of radioactive contamination. One difference between chemical pollution and radioactive contamination is that the chemical pollution is often visible, but radioactive contamination is unseen and deadly. We can see a factory or coal fired power plant smokestack spewing smoke. A river polluted with sewage and industrial waste is brown and sudsy. Radioactive contamination cannot be seen, but it has catastrophic and insidious effects.

Naturally occurring sources of radiation such as cosmic rays and minerals and stones like granite are external sources of radiation. Many man-made radiation sources are also external. X-rays in a hospital or dentists office are external. Workers in a nuclear power plant wear protective suits, but they still receive significant doses of external radiation.

> *Every person in the northern hemisphere today ... is continuously exposed to various types of low-level radiation.*

The atomic blast victims near ground zero at Hiroshima and Nagasaki received massive external doses of radiation, and scientists correlated their survival statistics with the amount of radiation that they received when the bombs exploded.

It is easy to measure and quantify the amount of external radiation we all receive in our environment. This is commonly done by the nuclear industry, and this data is used to "prove" that nuclear power is safe and that the amount of radiation that we receive from nuclear power is a tiny fraction of the naturally occurring background radiation.

But, the real danger from man-made nuclear contamination in our environment comes from "internal emitters" and not external radiation. Here is a good way to visualize the difference: Imagine that you are standing next to a wood-burning stove on a cold winter day. It is well stoked, practically glowing red, and you can feel the heat from it on your face and making your clothes hot. This is an example of external radiation. Its easy to measure. When you walk away from it your exposure to the heat stops. This is a key point with external radiation: the dose is controllable by changing your proximity to the source.

Now, imagine that this stove is fueled by magic wood, that burns intensely without needing air. Open the door, reach in with the fireplace shovel, scoop out some of the coals in a shovel and then smash them to a fine powder with a hammer. Next, take these finely powdered coals (which are still burning, they are magic) and inhale them, put them in your food and eat them and rub them all over your body. Each microscopic burning particle does not make enough heat to be measured, but its effects are felt by your cells right next to it.

This is exactly what is happening with man-made radioactive contamination in our environment. Due to the man-made sources of radiation mentioned earlier, every American and every person in the northern hemisphere today has radioactive particles lodged in their tissues and is continuously exposed to various types of low-level radiation. According to the outspoken British nuclear scientist Dr. Christopher Busby, "Internal radionuclides cannot be assessed by the current radiation risk model."

Ongoing low doses of radiation, over time, are devastating to health. The National Research Council's 2006 BEIR VII report states that there is no safe level of radiation exposure. This radiation amplifies the rates of all chronic degenerative diseases now found in human civilization, such as cancer, diabetes, heart disease and Alzheimer's. How does this happen? Particles of radionuclides stuck in our bodies constantly emit silent ionizing energy, which generates free radicals and breaks apart DNA. To quote Dr. Busby again: "Radiation does not just give you cancer, it increases the rate of just about every illness there is."

Starting in March 2011, the amount of man-made radioactive particles in our environment spiked upwards with the Fukushima power plant disaster. After the earthquake and tsunami, three reactors at this power plant melted down.

Three subsequent explosions (March 12th, 14th and 15th) released massive amounts of radioactive particles into the atmosphere. Due to the jet stream air currents, these particles blanketed the USA over the next few weeks. In addition, massive amounts of radionuclides have been released into the Pacific Ocean. An amount of radiation equal to the Chernobyl disaster was released after the first eleven days, and there are estimates that the total amount released over 20 years could exceed seven Chernobyls. In addition, Reactor 4 building still contains 1300 spent fuel rods. These could melt down if there is another large earthquake.

This amount of radiation is equal to 50 to 100 Chernobyls. According to a top nuclear operations expert, Arnold Gundersen of Fairewinds.org, "Fukushima is the biggest industrial catastrophe in the history of mankind."

What Can We Do?

Fortunately, there are steps that we can take to help prevent damage from this inevitable exposure to radioactive particles. We need to help our bodies excrete the particles that we have already inhaled or ingested. In addition, we need to flood our bodies with antioxidants and nutrients to neutralize free radicals and help regenerate and heal on a cellular level.

The regular consumption of miso products helps protect the body from some of the toxic effects associated with radioactivity.

Akizuki Diet

One of the first examples of how the proper diet could mitigate the effects of radiation occurred in Nagasaki, Japan after the atomic bomb blast. At the time of the atomic bombing, Tatsuichiro Akizuki, M.D. was Director of the Department of Internal Medicine at St. Francis's Hospital in Nagasaki and fed his staff and patients a strict diet of brown rice, miso and tamari soy soup, wakame, kombu and other seaweed, Hokkaido pumpkin, chinese cabbage, fresh fruits and sea salt. He prohibited the consumption of white flour, sugar and sweets. Sugars and sweets were forbidden because they suppress the immune system. Because of this diet he saved everyone in his hospital while many other survivors perished from the radiation sickness. Since this diet was low in calories, but rich in nutrients (high nutrient density), it helped to promote cellular repair through autophagy.

Another benefit of Akizuki's diet was the elimination of radionuclides through chelation and then elimination from the body. His diet contained chelating compounds from brown rice (phytates), seaweed (alginates), fruit (pectin), miso and cruciferous vegetables.

The regular consumption of miso products helps protect the body from some of the toxic effects associated with radioactivity exposure due to the presence of zybicolin and dipilocolonic acid, which act as binding agents (chelators) to detoxify and eliminate radioactive elements (such as strontium) and other pollutants from the body. Miso has been found to counteract the adverse effects of radiotherapy, chemotherapy, and environmental pollution.

The protective qualities of miso soup can be increased even more if ¼-ounce (5 grams) of dried kelp seaweed is added to the soup. Seaweed is able to neutralize radioactive isotopes in the human body because they bind to the sodium alginate in the seaweed and are excreted. However, given the current radioactive contamination in the ocean from Fukushima, be sure the seaweed is not from Japan.

Cruciferous Vegetables

Cruciferous vegetables (kale, cabbage, broccoli, etc.) contain isothiocyanates, compounds that bind to radionuclides present in foods—like Cesium 137, Strontium 90, and Cobalt 60—and prevent them from being absorbed into the body. In addition, isothiocyanates have been proven to be potent anti-cancer compounds.

The R.A.D. Regime

From our research we have come up with a regime using the highest grade Raw Antioxidants for Daily regeneration from the effects of radiation. We call this protocol the R.A.D. Regime, which consists of these powerhouse nutrient dense foods:

1. **Spirulina.** When disaster struck with the 1986 reactor meltdown at Chernobyl in the Ukraine, the neighboring state of Belarus was the most directly affected as winds were blowing north at the time. It received 70% of the radioactive fallout and 23% of its territory became contaminated with radioactivity. In total, over 160,000 children and hundreds of thousands of cleanup workers ("the Liquidators") became victims of radiation poisoning that produced higher incidents of birth defects, leukemia, anemia, cancers, thyroid disease, degeneration of spinal fluids, liver and bone marrow, and severely compromised immune systems.

   By taking 5 grams of spirulina a day for 45 days, the Institute of Radiation Medicine in Minsk found that the children showed enhanced immune systems and T-cell counts, and reduced radioactivity. The Institute also reported regeneration of bone marrow, spinal fluids, blood and the liver. Dangerously low white blood cell counts of about 1000, typical of leukemia, rose to an average of 3000 in 20 days, and the spirulina produced rapid improvements in the health of treated children compared to others who did not receive the algae.

   Spirulina reduced urine radioactivity levels by 50% in only 20 days' time and so the Institute developed a special program to treat 100 children every 20 days with spirulina. Health restoration was reported even when radiation sickness was so advanced that the children's eyeballs were bulging out of their sockets. The healing occurred even during the presence of radiation-contaminated food and water sources.

   Spirulina and other algae also contain high amounts of metallo-thionine compounds, which scientists think may strip the body of radioactive metals and protect against radiation damage. It also has a high content of chlorophyll and of beta-carotene that reduces free radical damage to cells and has even been used for treating cancer. (see **purehighlandliving.com**)

2. **Chlorella.** A natural wonder food. It is the most researched algae in the world, and many studies show it protects against radiation-induced chromosomal damage and has anti-tumor properties. In addition, chlorella builds the immune system, detoxifies heavy metals, normalizes blood sugar and blood

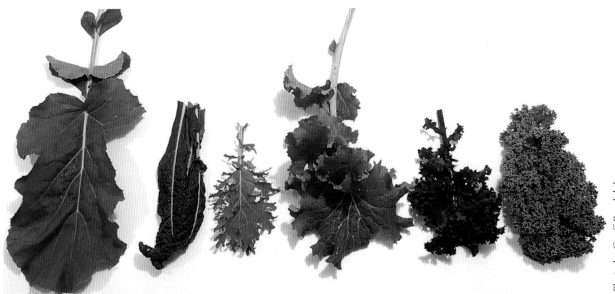

Six of the thirteen (!!) varieties of kale Geoff is growing.

pressure, balances the body's pH and fights cancer. Due to its extremely high chlorophyll content, it helps detoxify the liver, bowel and bloodstream.

Chlorella has the highest chlorophyll content of any known plant! It has 5–10 times the chlorophyll content of spirulina, wheat grass and barley grass. In addition to its chlorophyll content, chlorella's tough cell wall offers advantages not found elsewhere. When cracked via special processes, the cell wall has an outstanding surface area and ability to eliminate toxins, pesticides, and heavy metals from the body. Chlorella is an excellent eliminator of radioactive uranium, as the cellulose cell wall can bind with these particles and flush them out of the body.

Chlorella's cell wall also has the ability to induce interferon production, which helps with immune function (important during radiation sickness). Japanese doctors also discovered that giving chlorella to cancer patients going through radiation therapy helped prevent leucopenia, which is a sudden drop in your white blood cell count and a major problem with radiation illness. (USA: **phporder.com/ rawsome**)

3. **Vitamin C.** A well-known antioxidant that stimulates the body's enzyme systems responsible for neutralizing radiation exposure. Animal studies with hamsters and mice have proven Vitamin C's radiological protection. This is a widely available vitamin with a variety of health benefits, and there is no reason not to be taking it.

Our favorite source of natural Vitamin C is the Amla C Plus from Purium. This is an extract from the Amla berry, which is extensively used in Ayurvedic medicine. It is nature's best source of Vitamin C and is far superior to synthetic sources. (In the USA, order from: **phporder.com/rawsome**)

4. **Pectin and fiber.** One of the worst radionuclides contained in fallout is cesium-137. This element chemically mimics calcium, and is often found in high levels in milk, due to bio-accumulation. One of the best ways to remove cesium-137 contamination is with pectin. It binds with cesium in the gut and allows it to be easily excreted.

Children living in the parts of Belarus that are heavily contaminated by Chernobyl fallout have dangerously high levels of Cs-137 in their

bodies. There, researchers have given a 25-day pectin food additive treatment regime (5 gm. twice a day) to over 160,000 children. The results have demonstrated pectin's remarkable power. The level of Cs-137 in the children's organs decreased an average of 30 to 40% over each treatment.

5. **Astaxanthin.** One of the most powerful fat-soluble carotenoid antioxidants discovered is astaxanthin. Astaxanthin is extracted from marine algae, a natural carotenoid that gives salmon and egg yolks their characteristic color. Astaxanthin can physically improve the appearance of your skin and is 50 to 60 times better at free radical scavenging than vitamin C and beta-carotene. This is exactly what is needed to help repair radiation induced cellular oxidative damage and aid in the prevention of cancer cells.

Our favorite source of Astaxanthin is extracted from the Haematucoccus micro algae and is far superior to synthetic sources.*

6. **Melatonin.** Considered one of the most important tools for reversing radiation poisoning. It can help remove toxic metals such as Uranium, when taken with fiber and it has also been proven to be a major scavenger of pro-inflammatory oxygen- and nitrogen-based reactive molecules. It protects cells from the toxic effects of ionizing radiation, and promotes our immune response and regenerative repair.

The pineal gland generates melatonin during sleep, and it has been proven that nighttime melatonin generation is dramatically reduced by the blue spectrum present in artificial lighting. It is important to sleep in total darkness to enhance the natural production of melatonin during the night. Also, it is best if bright artificial lighting is restricted two hours before bedtime. Turn off the TV, computer and lights and break out the candles!

There are many brands of melatonin tablets available today, but most of them are synthetic melatonin. Our favorite source of natural melatonin (in addition to that which the body makes) is Apothe Cherry Concentrate from Purium Health Products. It is a concentrated extract of Montmorency tart cherries, and is an amazing natural source of the antioxidants melatonin, kaempferol and quercetin.*

7. **Zeolite.** In cases where the amounts of radioactive particles (especially Cesium-137) in the body are extremely high, the inorganic

zeolite minerals have been proven to be highly effective. Zeolites are micro-porous, crystalline minerals with unique well-defined structures. Because of their structure, zeolite molecules are one of the few negatively charged minerals in nature and they act like a magnet drawing toxins and heavy metals out of the body.

We prefer the Purium Health Products zeolite which is made from naturally occurring clinoptilolite. This particular type of zeolite has been used for over 800 years in traditional medicine to improve general health.*

*You can visit these websites to order the starred products:

USA: phporder.com/rawsome

UK: platinumuk.biz/rawsome

Summary

We could keep going with more supplements and therapies until you are so confused that you would not know where to start. However, the easy way to start is to eat miso soup with seaweed and cruciferous vegetables and supplement with chlorella and spirulina. As always, avoid wheat, flour, sweets and sugar. If you are living in an area where you suspect radiation contamination has occurred, then eating lower on the food chain is always a good idea. As more and more radiation from Fukushima flows into the Pacific Ocean, it may become prudent to avoid seafood caught there.

Sources

Fukushima Meltdown & Modern Radiation: Protecting Ourselves and Our Future Generations; John W. Apsley, Temet Nosce Publications, 2012.

How to Help Support the Body's Healing After Intense Radioactive or Radiation Exposure; Bill Bodri, Top Shape Publishing, LLC, 2004.

The Health Effects of Exposure to Uranium and Uranium Weapons Fallout; article by Christopher Busby, Documents of the European Committee on Radiation Risk No. 2 Brussels, 2010. **euradcom.org**

New Research Directions in DNA Repair, (Ch. 22: "Aspects of DNA Damage from Internal Radionuclides," article by Christopher Busby), InTech, 2013.

Radiation Dosimetry: Why Internal Emitters Are Different; article by Phillip Day, University of Manchester.

Dietary Practice of Hiroshima/Nagasaki Atomic Bomb Survivors; article by Hiroko Furo, Illinois Wesleyan University.

Report of the Committee Examining Radiation Risks of Internal Emitters (CERRIE), article by Dudley Goodhead et al. **cerrie.org**

Melatonin: an Established Antioxidant Worthy of Use in Clinical Trials; article by Ahmet Korkmaz et al, Molecular Medicine, January-February 2009

Surviving Radiation Exposure; article by Naoki Kubota.

Chapter III. Consequences of the Chernobyl Catastrophe for the Environment; Alexey V. Yablokov, Vassily B. Nesterenko, Alexey V. Nesterenko, Annals of the New York Academy of Sciences, Volume 1181.

Allyl isothiocyanate as a cancer chemopreventive phytochemical, article by Yuesheng Zhang, Molecular Nutrition & Food Research, January 2010.

Numbered references — see page 176.

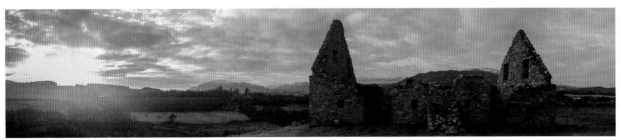

PURE Highland Living!

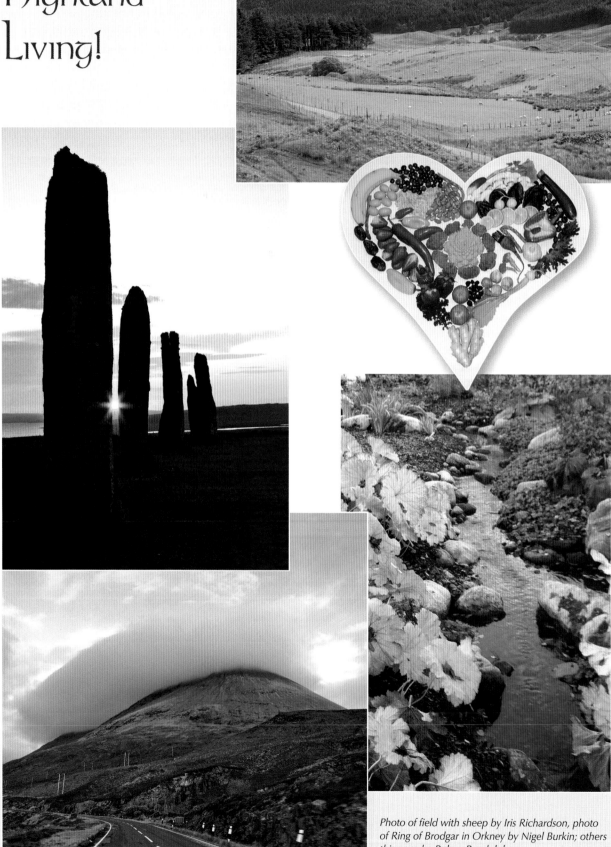

Photo of field with sheep by Iris Richardson, photo of Ring of Brodgar in Orkney by Nigel Burkin; others this page by Robyn Randolph.

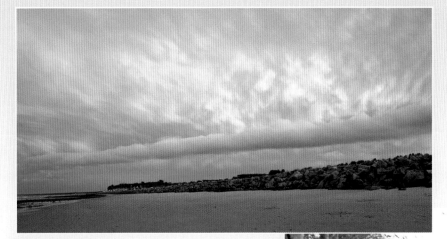

This is some of the landscape we have enjoyed while going around meeting and networking with other PURE, organic farmers and intuitive chefs in the highlands of Scotland.

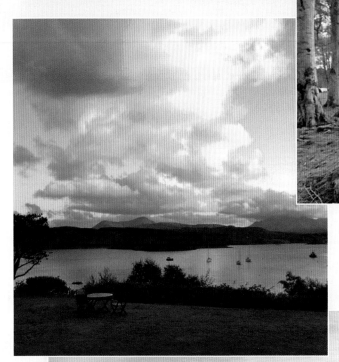

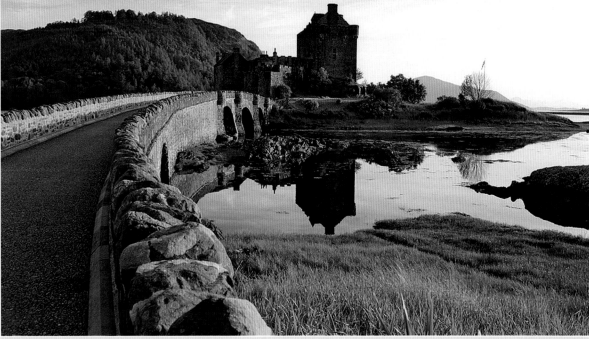

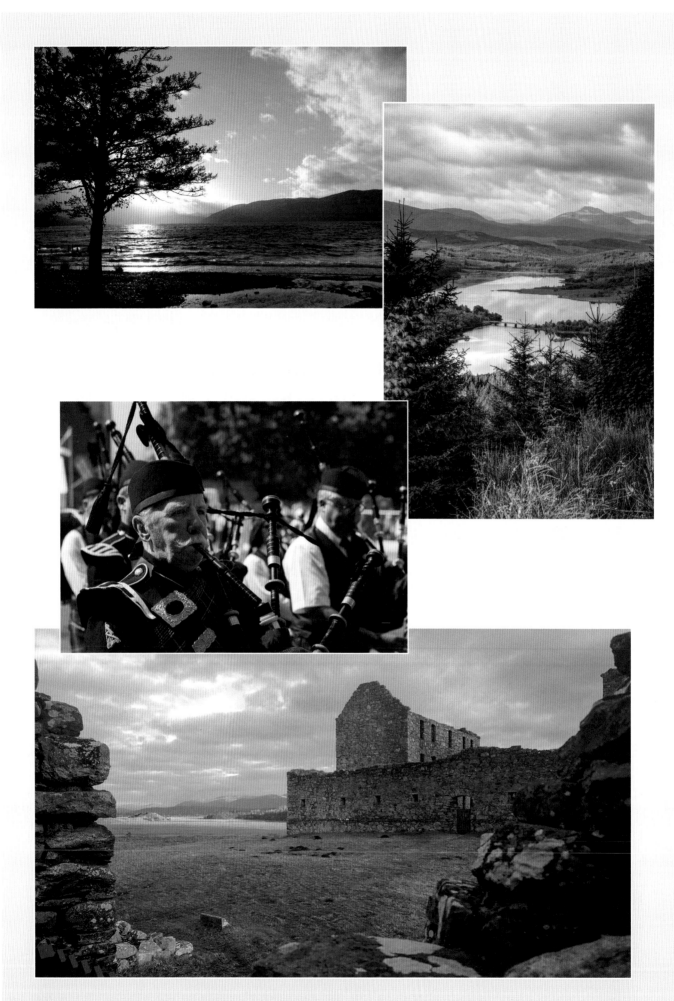

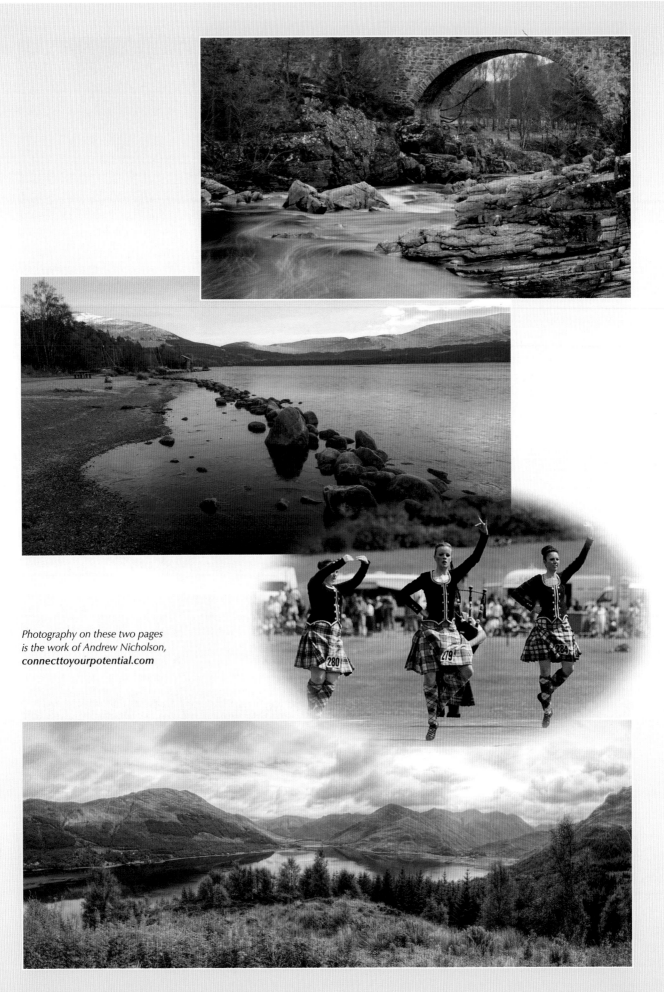

Photography on these two pages
is the work of Andrew Nicholson,
connecttoyourpotential.com

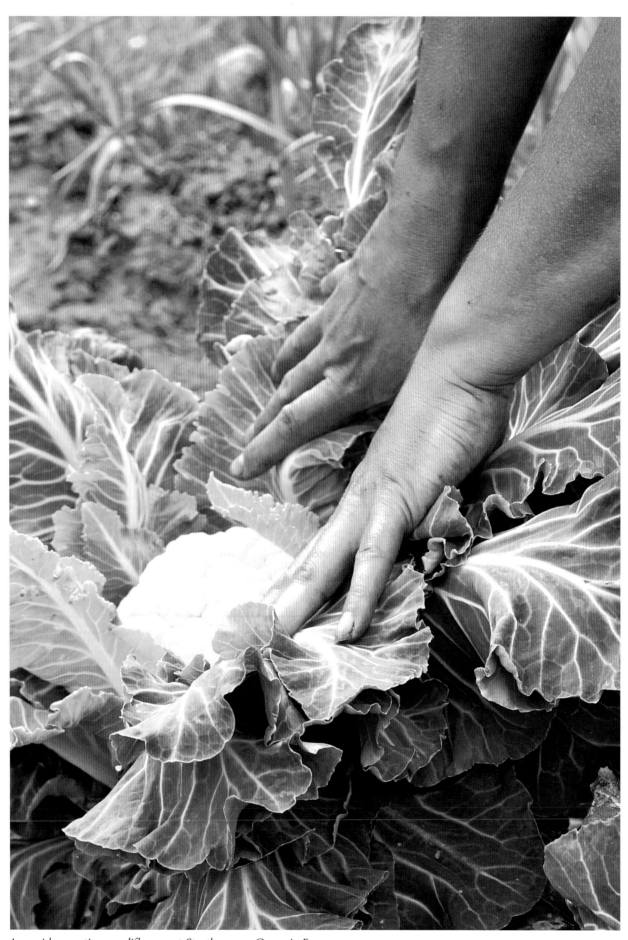

Jacqui harvesting cauliflower at Strathconan Organix Farm.

Nutrient Density is the Key to Successful Intermittent Fasting

Face it. During periods of calorie restriction on the "2 days" you will experience what may be a new feeling in your body. This is a feeling that we in the modern western world seldom feel. It's called: h-u-n-g-e-r. Yes. Did I really say that? I will say it again: HUNGER. There. I just said it again. When talking about food and diets, it seems as if hunger is the ultimate villain. Does the idea of hunger frighten you? It shouldn't!

For most of human existence, periodic hunger was a simple fact of life and people didn't go crazy from it or fear it any more than we today may fear getting sleepy or tired. It is simply a human biological response to a condition in our body.

What is different today is that most people in the western world are eating a highly refined, toxic diet based on manufactured foods made of processed grains, sugar and oils. When eating such a diet, the body no longer has the natural feedback and sensory mechanisms that it was designed to have with a PURE and healthy diet.

In 2010, Dr. Joel Fuhrman and a team of researchers conducted a fascinating study called "Changing perceptions of hunger on a high nutrient density diet."[26] In it, they compared in detail the changes in hunger feelings before and after adopting a high nutrient density diet. The "before" diet was a standard American/western diet (primarily a commercially processed food diet) with the majority of calories from sugars, white flour, refined oils, dairy and meat. The "after" diet was a high nutrient density combination of unrefined, unprocessed plant food with little added sugar and oils and a small amount of animal products. This diet was very high in micronutrients such as phytochemicals and antioxidants.

The results of this study have fascinating and crucial implications for successful intermittent fasting. They found that the frequency of "hunger pains" went from 80% often or more on the standard American/western diet to only 10%

...the frequency of "hunger pains" went from 80% or more on the standard American/Western diet to only 10% on the high nutrient density diet.

on the high nutrient density diet. If a meal was skipped, only 10% of the participants on the high nutrient density diet often or constantly felt discomfort. On the standard diet, over 70% of the participants, often or constantly felt discomfort after skipping a meal.

The study measured and compared the perceptions of hunger in many different ways, and the difference between the standard diet and the high nutrient density diet is dramatic in all comparisons. In addition to just feeling less hunger while eating a high nutrient density diet, the way that hunger actually impacted the participants was altered. When hungry, the participants eating a high nutrient density diet were actually less irritable and their moods were less affected. Hunger was no longer unpleasant.

When I first read this study, I thought, Eureka! This is indeed the Holy Grail of dieting! What good is a super healthy diet plan that has wonderful effects if you have to endure very unpleasant hunger all the time? Since you will be asking your body to effectively skip meals on the "2 days", we need a strategy to control the hunger and to prevent mood changes. Eating a high nutrient density diet will mitigate the experience of hunger and will allow you to endure the "2 days" with a feeling of control and pleasantness. Sensations such as fatigue, weakness, stomach cramps, irritability and headaches—which are commonly defined as hunger when eating the standard diet—are replaced by a new, less-unpleasant feeling of hunger when eating a high nutrient density diet. This is truly the key to making intermittent fasting feasible over the long term.

It is interesting to dig a bit deeper into the Fuhrman study and read about the reasons why there is this difference in perceived hunger for the two different diets. When eating a standard American/western diet that is low in antioxidant and phytochemical micronutrients, there is a buildup of toxins and inflammatory by-products. When digestion ceases between meals, there are actually the physical symptoms of withdrawal. These symptoms Fuhrman calls "toxic hunger." He also notes that these withdrawal symptoms drive overeating and are a major factor leading to obesity.

In the attempt to avoid these withdrawal/hunger symptoms that result from the standard diet, people often become trapped in an endless cycle of continuous digestion, frequent eating and excessive caloric intake. Overweight and obese people eating the standard diet often only feel "normal" when eating too frequently. As noted by Popkin and Duffey,[26] there has been a dramatic increase in the frequency of "eating occasions" over the last 30 years in the USA. The average adult eating occasion was 3.5 per day in 1977. This rose to 5.0 per day in 2006. From 1977 to 2006, the time between eating occasions dropped from 4.5 hours to 3.5 hours and the average adult calories consumed rose from 2090 to 2533.

This study shows that by eating a diet of toxic industrial food, we have lost our ability to feel our body telling us how much food we actually need. Consequently, there is an increased tendency to eat all the time, even when there is no real need for calories.

Other researchers in different studies have confirmed the findings made by Fuhrman. In a study by researchers at Penn State University, 71 obese women were put on a reduced fat diet to lose weight.[27] They were allowed to eat all of the food that they wanted (*ad libitum*), but to focus on reducing the energy density of their diets by reducing the fat ratio. The group was split into two, and one of the groups were also instructed to increase the water-containing food content by eating all of the fresh fruit and vegetables that they wanted. This is the basic definition of a high nutrient density diet.

After one year, both groups had lost significant amounts of weight. The group that only reduced the fat content of their diet had lost an average of 14 pounds, and the group that also incorporated more fruit and vegetables into their diets lost an average of 17 pounds. Due to the reduced energy density of the water rich fruit and vegetables, the second group actually ate 25% more food by weight. But, the really interesting outcome from the study was related to hunger. The increased fruit and vegetable group reported less hunger.

The researchers observed that in other clinical trials, hunger has been linked with the lack of weight loss and weight regain. Also, it was noted that a dietary strategy that helps with the control of hunger through the increased mass of food eaten, helps lead to more weight loss.

We assert, and the philosophy of PURE 5:2 is, that in order to do Intermittent Fasting for the best possible results, one must eat high nutrient density foods (like kale, spirulina, barely grass, chlorella,

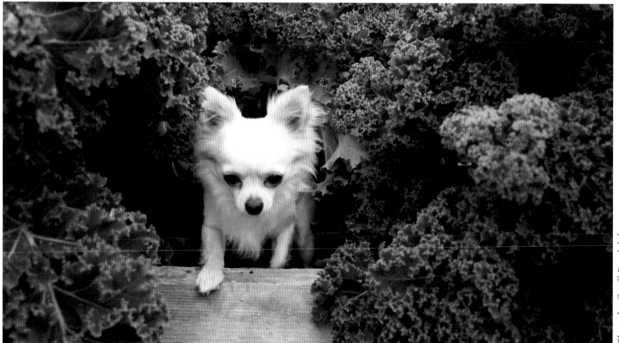

Our dog Harry, romping in the gigantic kale leaves in our raised beds. Learn to grow your own kale, then make raw kale salads or kale chips to snack on!

etc.) while avoiding barren, toxic and low nutrient density foods. Certain foods will create havoc with the body's metabolic system, interrupting the normal feedback that our body gives us and making it nearly impossible to endure any level of fasting. The worst foods are processed foods, especially those containing sugar and/or high glycemic index ingredients such as white flour. Eating these foods has the effect of spiking the blood sugar levels, which causes the pancreas to overcompensate and release too much insulin. This, in turn, causes the blood sugar to crash and creates a strong hunger and desire to eat more sugar to raise the blood sugar again. This nasty cycle can be avoided by eating pure unrefined foods that digest slowly and do not cause the blood sugar to spike.

What are the implications for intermittent fasting? If you want to be successful at intermittent fasting, then one of the primary real life concerns is controlling your feelings of hunger, especially during the fast days. Research clearly shows that the best way to do this is to eat a high nutrient density diet including fruits and vegetables that contain plenty of water and the micronutrients needed to detoxify the body. Also key is nutrient dense food that digests slowly so as to avoid blood sugar spikes and drops. This exactly describes the PURE 5:2 diet, which is discussed in the following chapters.

About Weight Loss – Don't Gain or Lose Weight by Losing Your Health!

Excess weight is a sign of dis-ease in the body. It is a symptom that the body is not able to properly handle what is ingested. There are usually several factors involved such as excessive food intake, poor food metabolism, toxic and chemical foods that drag the system down, lack of exercise, blood sugar issues, etc. No matter what the combination of circumstances that led to weight gain, for weight loss to be significant, permanent and healthy, several factors must exist.

First and foremost, the body must be detoxified. Years of old toxins are stored in the fat cells. When we ingest foods loaded with preservatives and chemicals, our bodies don't know how to relate to these foreign substances. They aren't like proteins, carbohydrates or fats, so the body either treats them as invaders and works very hard to process and filter them out, or instead these poisons are stored in fat cells. In fact the body manufactures fatty pockets (out of fat cells) to warehouse these peculiar substances. The result of this is very odd-shaped, flabby cellulite bodies that possess fatty rolls to house these unhealthy toxins. Elimination of toxins and the breaking down of fat cells is the key to success. This is where eating lots of raw and PURE foods come in. There are some specific foods that we use to help the

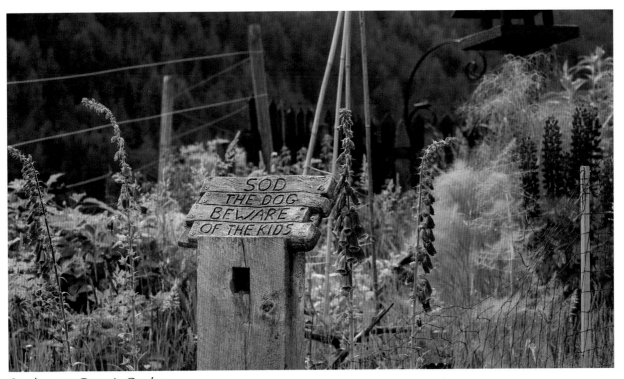

Strathconan Organix Garden

body detox to provide the body with the correct components that grease the wheels, so to speak. With the permission of David Sandoval, C.E.O. of Purium Health Products and author of *The Green Foods Bible*, here is a portion of a tape lecture he gave concerning the value of green foods, which expands on what I am saying:

"Now, many people talk about the need to eliminate properly and they discuss fiber. But did you know that we need potassium and cell salts in order to create an environment that eliminates toxins from the body? You see, potassium causes the bowel to contract and sodium causes the bowel to expand. So, when you take green foods, which create abundant potassium and cell salts in the environment where the intestines contract and expand, then proper elimination can take place. If we only take fiber as a means of increasing our elimination, then we can actually suffer by bulking up and bulking up and literally stretching the bowel, stretching the skin of the intestines. It is only through eating these green foods that have both potassium and cell salts that we create the environment of contraction and expanding that leads to proper elimination on a daily basis of accumulated waste in the bowel; so it's not just fiber, it is also trace minerals which lead to proper elimination."

"Drinking plenty of purified water gives the body a way to eliminate old toxic material. Next, cravings have to be addressed. Adding foods rich in chromium can help decrease food cravings. Foods such as brewer's yeast, apples, whole grains and some seafood can make an impact. Drinking green drinks as well as fresh vegetable juices can provide much needed cell nutrition, offering the body vital nutrients it has been starving for. Once these nutrients are delivered, the cravings quiet down tremendously.

"By eating vitamin and mineral-rich complex carbohydrates, continual hunger can be curtailed. Often when people start eating a mostly raw diet they find that their hunger vanishes and they experience a new sense of being nourished, which leads to eating satisfaction.

Often when people start eating a mostly raw diet they find that their hunger vanishes and they experience a new sense of being nourished.

"As we get older, the issue of metabolism intensifies! We have to find ways to take in foods that our bodies can process, use and burn in the most efficient way. When our bodies are burdened or not able to digest food properly, this can cause various metabolic processes that can lead to weight gain. Exercise plays an important role in metabolism as well as providing a way to encourage the body to work synergistically to eliminate toxins and waste materials.

"Paying close attention to foods that cause reactions and eliminating those foods will greatly increase your ability to be successful. One way to perceive food sensitivity is to take your pulse prior to eating and then 30, 60 and 90 minutes later. Keeping a food journal, tracking all foods eaten daily, and documenting any altered pulse rates can be a tremendous tool for getting a grasp on what is working and what isn't."

The below information is edited, with permission from *Power Health with Spirulina—Nature's Richest Whole Food*, an educational guide by Pure Planet Products, Inc. (makers of my favorite carob mint spirulina):

"Losing weight, or more specifically, body fat, can be a source of frustration to those changing their eating habits. This is largely due to a lack of knowledge about body chemistry, and the various ways the body stores and uses nutrition, especially as it relates to the accumulation, use and storage of fat.

"Though decreasing food intake may lower overall weight, cutting calories alone does not maintain muscle tissue nor does it reverse the altered chemistry of the muscles, nor does it permanently keep the body from resuming its previous fat set point. In fact, a weight loss quick-fix attacks subcutaneous fat first and will remove intramuscular fat only under the most severe circumstances. To instruct the body to undergo such rigor would be disappointing at best because nothing prevents weight gain once again. Radical dieting, unbalanced eating, shots and prolonged fasting can worsen the situation because they have been shown to lessen muscle mass as the person is losing fat.

"How does the body respond to all of this? The body's first reaction is to draw on the energy that is immediately available in any emergency. This is not fat; the body has no means to make immediate use of stored fat. The body's immediately available form of energy is glycogen which is a form of glucose (a carbohydrate) stored with water in the muscles and in the body's most metabolically active vital organ, the liver.

"For many years it was assumed that the glycogen stored in the liver was the principal source of blood sugar between meals. However, more recently it has been shown that the liver hoards this glycogen. Instead of giving up its glycogen for blood sugar, the liver converts protein to glucose. This means that if the body were to subsist on a starvation diet, it would actually convert valuable body protein to blood sugar as fuel for the brain.

"Spirulina is the only plant food that contains glycogen. Glycogen is not ordinarily available through our diet. Muscles store glycogen and use it as a principal source of both immediate and long-term energy. The more glycogen available during intense or sustained exercise, the greater the potential for improved functioning. When glycogen levels drop,

weakness and fatigue set in rapidly. Spirulina shortcuts the metabolic process of synthesizing glycogen from our food and supplies it directly, pre-formed, thus sparing the body's own glycogen reserves.

"The amount of fat that we might gain is not genetically pre-ordained, but determined by our chosen lifestyles. When a person reaches adult weight, the body establishes the enzyme system, hormone levels, and musculoskeletal pattern to remain at that weight. Whatever amount of fat one maintains for a period of a year or more then becomes the body's reference point. From then on all body systems will be geared to that reference or fat set point. The body protects its fat cells against invasion and deprivation just as it protects all other cells, so if overweight for a year or more, the body demands to be kept at this set point.

"Exercise is a key component that can successfully help reset the body's set point. Daily exercise, such as aerobic, brisk walking, where the lungs are breathing deeply and the heart is working vigorously, forms a central part of permanent fat loss. This is true for two major reasons: first, regular aerobic exercise

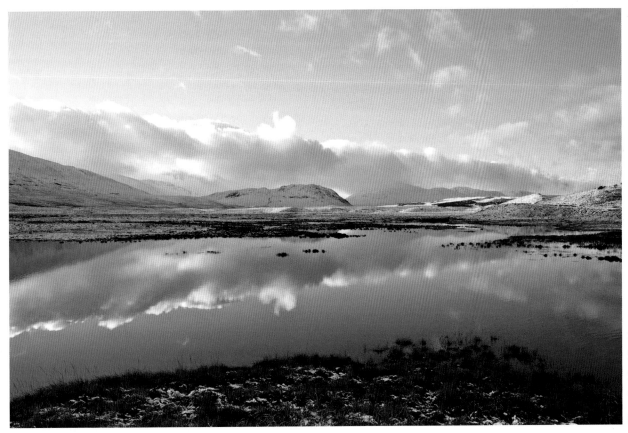

The gorgeous hills of Loch Laggan in the Scottish Highlands.

stimulates metabolism, which in itself helps burn fat, and second, such exercise encourages the rapid and efficient elimination of toxicity from the system through the breath, the skin (in the form of sweat), the bowels and the kidneys. It even improves the functions of the liver, which is absolutely central to solving the problem of excess fat-stores in the body.

"A key factor to explain why some people lose weight while some seem to maintain normal weight effortlessly is the efficiency of special tissue in the back of the neck and along the spine, called brown adipose tissue or brown fat. Unlike ordinary yellow fat, brown fat has a very high metabolic response to any excess calories consumed, by burning them off as body heat rather than storing them as fat. Unfortunately, many overweight people suffer from under-active brown fat.

Discovering spirulina and learning how to use it can awaken a deeper interest in a more natural diet through its powerful rejuvenating effects.

"A number of factors are known to contribute to the activation of brown fat. Interestingly, the essential fatty acid (EFA) content of body fat is inversely proportional to body weight. This means that the higher the level of EFAs in the body, the lower the body weight, and vice versa.

"At the University of Wales in Cardiff, studies indicate that gamma linoleic acid (GLA) has a stimulating effect on brown fat tissue. The prostaglandins, which are the end products of GLA metabolism, possibly accelerate the mitochondria activity of the brown fat. There is no better food source of GLA readily available than spirulina.

"Spirulina also contains phenylalanine, which is a natural appetite suppressant. Phenylalanine, an amino acid, produces a chemical known as cholecystokinin, which in turn acts quickly on the appetite center of the hypothalamus in the brain. This helps suppress appetite. Spirulina is one of the most easily assimilated forms of protein, keeping blood sugar at the correct level and preventing hunger pangs. Taking six to ten tablets of 100% pure spirulina on an empty stomach one half hour before meals is an effective and beneficial method for weight loss.

"Spirulina is an exceptionally rich source of arginine, an amino acid that releases growth hormone (Gh). Gh is a polypeptide hormone that is secreted by the pituitary gland. Gh stimulates the body's own regenerative process by increasing the rate of protein synthesis. It causes muscle cells to grow and multiply by directly increasing the rate at which amino acids enter the muscles and are built up into protein. Gh promotes fat burning, causing cells to switch from burning carbohydrates to burning fat for energy. It stimulates fat tissues to release stored fat and it stimulates other cells to break down the released fat molecules.

"With a desire to decrease body fat, one must increase lean muscle tissue and muscle enzymes through exercising and ensuring that the diet contains branched chain amino acids (BCAAs) for muscle biosynthesis. Three BCAAs, leucine, isoleucine and valine, provide more than 70% of all the free nitrogen to the body and regulate muscle protein synthesis. Even if one is sedentary, the muscles burn 90% of all the calories burned. Specialized enzymes existing only in muscle tissue can increase fat burning by fifty-fold during exercise. Eating the three BCAAs will supply fuel and be converted into glucose for energy when you have high energy demands and diminishing blood sugar levels. If dietary BCAAs are lacking, the body will break down its own muscle tissue resulting in loss of lean muscle mass, lowered metabolism and increased fat deposition.

"Spirulina is nature's richest source of BCAAs. It is important to eat as much live or biogenic food as possible. The word biogenic means life-generating, and it refers to living, enzyme-rich, raw foods. Living foods have special properties for both weight loss and high-level health. Fresh fruits (organic whenever possible), sprouted seeds and grains have the highest complement of vitamins and minerals, essential fatty acids, easily assimilated top quality protein, fiber and wholesome carbohydrates. Such a natural complement of nutrients in superbly balanced form supplies the body with substances it needs to function at a high level of efficiency. This is what one wants in order to encourage steady and permanent fat loss.

"Discovering spirulina and learning how to use it can awaken a deeper interest in a more natural diet through its powerful rejuvenating effects. Its super nutrition satisfies hunger because it completely meets the body's biochemical needs.

"The use of spirulina can help re-establish normal sodium/potassium and acid/alkaline balance. Excess fat and water are reduced, returning the body to a leaner, better balance. The change is gentle, indirect and stable."

NOTE: For the spirulinas we recommend, see our websites as noted in Chapter 6, *Get Equipped.*

All Proteins Are Not Created Equal

There are nine essential amino acids that make up a complete protein. Rice and beans for example eaten on their own do not make a complete protein yet they do when eaten together. Typically we have been taught to count how many grams of protein are in a food and told to eat protein in terms of amounts of grams.

As it is true that not all calories provide the same type of fuel, the same can be said about the grams of proteins. Further, it is not the quantity that counts but the quality. In the case of proteins we must learn to assess the balance of the amino acids over the amount of grams of actual protein.

There is a lot of misinformation about protein and how much and what type we require. Beef, for example, contains eleven amino acids. Of those eleven, four comprise the bulk, making the protein very unbalanced. Ideally the best form of protein is one where there are at least nine amino acids that are weighted very evenly. The best example of a balanced, perfect protein is really from a plant-based food, not from cattle as the meat industry would lead you to believe.

Spirulina and chlorella (from algae) are examples of the best protein sources because they are made up of all nine essential amino acids and additionally they are balanced in a natural ratio to one another. Most animal proteins are heavily weighted in some of the amino acids while significantly lower in others.[28]

The highest percentage of protein found in any whole food is 60% found in spirulina and chlorella. The body thrives on this food because of the broad array of amino acids in the correct proportion to one another. Even wheat grass is only 24% protein in comparison, yet comes in higher in balanced protein content than meat. Meat actually is about 25% protein, whereas kale

and broccoli can boast 45% protein content. Cooked meat also provides no enzymes and tends to make the body more acidic. These are two additional important reasons to choose plant-based protein sources such as spirulina and chlorella as a higher density nutritional form of protein.

The right type of protein aids proper food digestion and is a catalyst for nutrients to be efficiently extracted and absorbed by the body. To ensure proper digestion, only 2–4 grams of either spirulina or chlorella is needed to go along with other foods. Consider adding spirulina or chlorella with every meal. Purium Health Products makes a carob mint spirulina (the carob mint makes it way more palatable this way) tablet that is chewable and great to have right before a meal.

The Right Fats Don't Make You Fat, Carbs Do!

One of the most effective ways to help you reach and maintain a healthy weight is to eliminate the wrong kind of carbs found in grains and especially in wheat. According to a new study, revealed at The Endocrine Society's 93rd Annual Meeting, even a moderate reduction in carbohydrate-rich foods can produces less deep body fat (intra-abdominal fat). This is the type of fat that has been linked to type 2 diabetes, stroke and heart disease.

There is no doubt with all the current research that one of the biggest blunders, if not the biggest in all of diet and health history, was the push for lowfat eating. Eating healthy fat does NOT make you fat. Carbohydrates from sugars and grains do! When people were convinced fats were bad, especially butter, they turned to processed and sugar loaded carbohydrates to fill the void. Fats eaten in the proper balance and the right types actually aid the pancreas in slowing down the spikes in blood sugar when eating carbs.

Without the proper fats in the diet, a great imbalance has occurred, resulting in a horrific disturbance in homeostasis in the body. The imbalance of fat to sugar ratio is at the crux of diabetes. This has created an epidemic that now affects innocent children as well as adults. The message needs to go far and wide about the dangers of eating low fat and especially artificial fat products like margarines and butter-like substitutes.

Finding blood sugar balance has been a life-long pursuit for me, unlike Geoff who is much more able to do high-intensity workouts in a fasting state. The brainwashing about eating fat seems to have seeped into every fiber of my being. It is as if someone gave me the "get out of jail card" for free, after a lifetime of captivity. I can't believe the door is open and I can walk forward, no longer a captive of that thinking. It just seems too good to be true to be able to eat butter with no guilt. I have bought the lie my whole life, and it is taking a while to sink in.

Every day you cast your vote by the foods you buy and the restaurants you pay money to support. Be a part of the food and health revolution and spend your money supporting those who support healthy and safe eating practices. Realize any processed food made in a factory represents foods that tear your body down rather than build it up.

The first place to start with the out-of-control obesity problem is simply to eliminate unhealthy carbs in the form of grains (especially processed grains) and sugar (in its various forms and especially anything comprised of high-fructose corn syrup) and replace that with more healthy fats.

According to Dr. Mercola, of **mercola.com**, "The ideal ratio between carbs, fats and protein depends on your nutritional type. We all need some fat, but some of us need upwards of 50% of our diet in the form of fat, while others need as little as 10%. The ideal ratio depends on your nutritional type."

We agree with Dr. Mercola that there is not one type of diet for everyone. We are all unique with a wide range of variables that play into how we digest the amount and type of calories we consume. If you are interested in understanding more about what nutritional type you are so you can zero in on what foods and in what ratios are the best for your metabolism, you can take Mercola's free test online at: **products.mercola.com/nutritional-typing/**

When I took his test I found it was a confirmation of what I already intuitively understood. See how much you intuitively already know about yourself by looking over the different nutritional types prior to taking the test. See if you already know what your type is just by tuning into yourself intuitively! (That is an excellent way to exercise and develop you intuitive muscle!)

The next place to go with the out-of-control obesity problem (once you intuitively zero in on the right ratio for you) is to begin to include more healthy fat in your diet such as: coconut oil, olive oil, animal-based fats (grass-fed meats, omega-3 fish oils, and raw dairy products), nuts, seeds, and avocados. Remove all fats from highly refined sources (trans fats and hydrogenated).

When you learn your nutritional type, you don't have to worry about counting calories or fat grams ever again. Instead focus on eating the

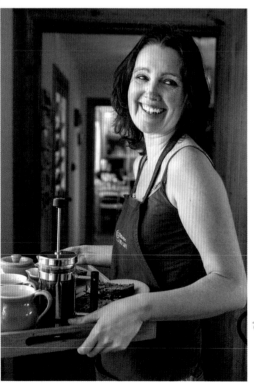

Support restaurants like Ellishader Art Cafe in Staffin, Skye who use local, organic ingredients in their food!

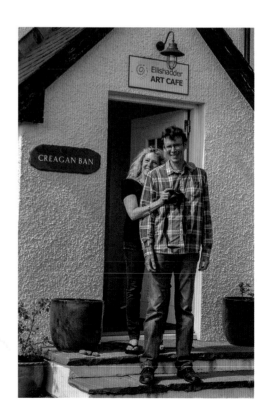

right proportion of carbs, fats and protein for your unique body and circumstances.

There are particular types of fats known as MUFA (which stands for monounsaturated fatty acid) that have gained popularity with regards to helping reduce belly fat. Studies have shown that including one serving of MUFA with every meal can help with weight loss without cutting calories. MUFAs provide other healthy benefits as well, such as helping to control type 2 diabetes, reducing the risk of heart disease and reducing the markers of inflammation.

Eating PURE Foods to Reverse Insulin Resistance and Diabetes

Like many people today, I was raised eating a high-processed carbohydrate diet. I have always had blood sugar issues until I started eating mostly raw foods. I remember passing out when I was ten and cutting my head open from low blood sugar. Having had my father die from diabetes keeps me on my toes striving to see over the diabetes horizon into a new vista that could be possible if we heed the warnings and take on the solutions. I realized again, recently, that my cholesterol seems to suggest possible insulin resistance and learned from my friend Mary Toscano, author of *Sweet Fire*, how much genetics play a part in the diabetes equation. As we wrote this book, we, too find areas where we need to tighten our belts and regroup. Eating PURE and taking the best care of ourselves is an ongoing process.

For those with blood sugar issues, insulin resistance and diabetes, it is important to pay attention to the GI (Glycemic Index) of foods as well as the relatively new understanding of GL (Glycemic Load).

GI is a number given to a food, relative to that of glucose, which represents that food's ability to increase the level of glucose in the blood. The higher the number, the greater the blood sugar response or spike. A GI of 70 or more is high, a GI of 56 to 69 is medium, and a GI of 55 or less is low.

GI refers to the quantity not the quality of the carbohydrates. Not all carbohydrates act the same in the body. High on the GI scale are foods that

are quickly broken down in the intestines with the result of rapidly rising blood glucose levels.

For the most part, low-glycemic foods are fiber-rich foods and seem to have less effect on blood sugars. Potatoes are an example of a high-glycemic index food. The effect of potatoes on blood sugar actually is higher than that of sucrose (table sugar).

Determining what works best in each person's body may require a bit of work. Important factors to consider include age and activity level, the amount of fiber and fat in the particular food, how refined (processed) the food is, what else was eaten with the food, what the composition of the food is in terms of carbohydrates, protein and fat, how the food was cooked, and how quickly your body digests the food (which varies from person to person).

Whereas GI tells you how rapidly a particular carbohydrate turns into sugar, the GL completes the picture by telling you how much of that carbohydrate is in a serving of a particular food.

You need to know both things to understand a food's effect on blood sugar. For example, a piece of watermelon has a high GI of 72, but its carbohydrate content is only 5%. Therefore you take the GI of 72 and multiply by 5% and it gives you 3.6, which is the GL. GL greater than 20 is considered high, 11–19 medium, 10 or less is low.

To study this further and see excellent food charts showing GI and GL scores go to: **mendosa.com/ gilists.htm**

Even if you are not aware of having blood sugar issues, chances are good that if you eat a traditional western diet you have some form of blood sugar spiking going on.

Who is at risk?

Everyone who lives and breathes needs to be concerned about hypoglycemia and diabetes. Energy is produced from glucose, and glucose is produced from our food. If we are not eating properly, we are not producing efficient energy. Then we begin storing fat, and we set the stage for illness and disease. Any time one of our basic needs is out of balance, the body is under stress and cannot function properly.

Pop Quiz: Answer True or False

1. **A potato processes slower than sucrose (table sugar) in your body.**

2. **Instant brown rice breaks down into sugar slower than beans.**

3. **White bread breaks down into sugar slower than fruit.**

If you answered false to all three questions then you are correct!

Most people walk around every day in some state of blood sugar imbalance. The symptoms of hypoglycemia and diabetes are a clear indication that the body is not processing or metabolizing glucose properly. The most overlooked symptoms are fatigue, depression, stress and obesity. There is a direct correlation between obesity and insulin insensitivity. However, you do not have to be 50 to 100 lbs. overweight to have blood sugar problems. If you are overweight, you have a 200% greater chance of developing Type II diabetes, which usually manifests itself with hypoglycemia first. Left undiagnosed, untreated and unmanaged, hypoglycemia can turn into diabetes.

Symptoms:

Feeling shaky, sweating, dizziness, weakness and/or overwhelming tiredness, rapid heartbeat, numbness or tingling in mouth or lips, hunger

Other symptoms that may come on more slowly are:

Crying, irritability and/or anger, drowsiness, mental confusion and/or difficulty in thinking, poor coordination (may result in trouble walking), blurred vision and/or headaches, slurred speech.

If you are currently experiencing these symptoms, it is important to consult your doctor before attempting fasting. Your first priority is to understand how to eat the correct balance of PURE foods for your metabolism. You may need to modify what we are suggesting for the PURE 5:2 transformation, as this is not the best approach for everyone, especially those with blood sugar issues. Take it easy and be careful if you have any blood sugar issues and do seek trained professional help.

Because I tend to have insulin sensitivity on my "2" days I have a green smoothie around 10 am, after warm lemon water. Then in the afternoon I will make fresh juice and add a heaping tablespoon of coconut oil to help balance the sugars in the carrot juice. Geoff will tend to go all day without needing much and from time to time snack on leaves of kale or pieces of broccoli. My metabolism is a bit different. Whereas he can do strenuous kettle bell workouts on "2" days, I prefer gentle yoga stretching.

We are all different and need to intuitively find what works best for our own unique bodies.

PURE Food and Balance For Hypoglycemic Help

1. High-protein Foods

Foods such as lean cuts of grass fed beef, lamb, turkey, chicken, eggs and nuts are high in protein. The best form of plant protein comes from spirulina. High-protein foods take time to digest and break down slowly in the body, which helps to keep blood sugar levels stable. Keep in mind that the best proteins are those with a balance of amino acids, as this is more important than the actual grams of protein. In other words, it is the quality of the protein that matters when it comes to metabolizing the protein. Spirulina is our favorite choice as it contains approximately 70% protein by weight. Be sure to pick a source that is not coming from radiation-contaminated waters (since Fukushima).

2. Complex Carbohydrates

Complex carbohydrates include tubers and vegetables. These foods are digested more slowly than simple carbohydrates like white flour, sugar and processed foods.

3. High-fiber Foods

Soluble-fiber foods are a must for those with blood sugar issues, helping prevent rapid blood sugar spikes by slowing down the rate at which sugar enters the bloodstream. Consistent, steady, sustained energy is the goal and soluble fiber will help to take you there. Be sure to incorporate foods like garbanzo and kidney beans into soups and salads. Use oat groats (the best choice for oats as it contains the entire grain except for the inedible outer hull) to replace rice and other grains. Most fruit and vegetables contain fiber. Lima beans, artichokes, spinach, broccoli, carrots, apples and flax seeds are particularly high in soluble fiber. Mix blueberries with cinnamon and vanilla for a high-antioxidant, soluble-fiber snack.

4. Healthy Fats

Eating a moderate amount of healthy fats with your meals and snacks will help to prevent spikes and subsequent falls in blood sugar. Choose monounsaturated and polyunsaturated fats such as avocados, olive oil and nut butters.

Both soluble and insoluble fiber play an important role in maintaining health.

5. Lemon and Apple Cider Vinegar to the Rescue

Lemon juice helps slow digestion, and apple cider vinegar proved its merit in a 2007 study showing two tablespoons of vinegar diluted in water taken at bedtime lowered glucose levels by morning by 4–6%. (Note: not recommended for diabetics as apple cider vinegar contains chromium, which can alter insulin levels). Use vinegar in salad dressings. Lemon can be used in water and salad dressings as well.

When it comes to hypoglycemia think balance, balance, balance — and then think balance some more! It's all about keeping the balance and not spiking up only to crash down. Balance. The best management of hypoglycemic symptoms is maintaining a balanced diet that includes all of these food groups, in the right proportions. Intuitively find your balance somewhere in the range of 35 to 45% complex carbohydrates, 25 to 35% protein, and 25 to 35% fat. Keep to this ratio for every meal and snack that you consume throughout the day. This will help you balance out. Once you find your balance for a few months… then you can slowly and intuitively progress with PURE 5:2. Take your time. Go slow and move forward with your best health and nutrition in mind.

The key to anti-aging involves eating nutrient-dense foods, loaded with enzymes, in such a way

When it comes to hypoglycemia think balance, balance, balance — and then think balance some more!

as to keep your insulin levels as consistently low as possible.

Applying the nutritional type and GI/GL information to the PURE 5:2 Transformation will yield the very best natural, intuitive way of eating. You will know when you find the right ratio for you because you will feel balanced, clear-headed and with wonderful, even, energy and vitality! This is what healthy eating and living is all about!

The Addiction to Sugar and Grains

Walk through a typical supermarket today and look at the food that we really eat in our Westernized diet. One way to categorize the foods is to look at how many of them contain either sugar or some form of grains. Usually the grains will have been processed in some form. Probably 60% or more of the Western diet is made up of these items.

Grains and sugars form the backbone of the modern industrialized food system. They are the universal building blocks of manufactured foods, along with denatured seed oils such as

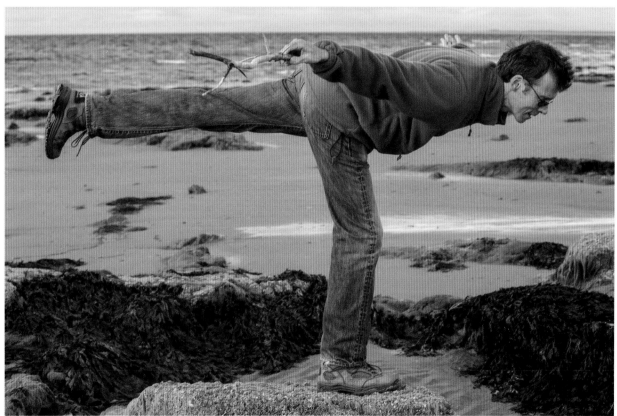

It's all about balance...

Photo by Robyn Randolph

safflower or cottonseed oils. Think about it from the perspective of a food factory owner. With the right combinations of cheap oils, cheap sugar (HFCS), flour, salt, and artificial flavorings, you can create an endless combination of food-like substances. Then, all it takes is the right branding, promotion, and marketing and you can create new products like breakfast cereals, toaster pops, bread, biscuits, crackers, cookies, candies, and so on. You could even brand some of these items "healthy" and call them energy bars, breakfast bars, protein bars, rice cakes, or heart-healthy whole grain whatevers. How do the supermarkets even keep up with all of these new "food-like" creations that appear each year?

It's a dream for manufacturers, as they have the ingredients to keep creating ever more new food-like substances. Items that never existed in nature now are a branded commodity that every person can recognize. This is further proof that the rules of capitalism are not the rules of health!

Sugar: Villain #1

Cutting sugar out of my diet has always seemed like a no-brainer. Everyone knows that sugar is bad for you. Yes, yes, I know. Sugar is bad. I knew this. But, I didn't always practice it. The question is do you really believe it enough to be willing to swim against the strong currents in our Western culture and actually choose to eliminate sugar from your diet? There are some excellent videos you can watch on YouTube, by Dr. Robert Lustig and others, that will completely change the way that you look at sugar. Take an hour or two to watch them and you will forever change the way you look at a "harmless" bite of sweets.

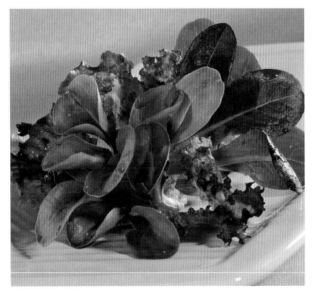

You can never eat too much fresh greens!

Sugar is highly addictive and can:

1. lead to hypoglycemia and insulin resistance
2. promote inflammation in the body
3. fuel cancer to thrive
4. lead to weight gain
5. contribute to non-alcoholic fatty liver disease
6. suppress immune system
7. reduce high-density lipoproteins (HDL)
8. cause mineral deficiencies
9. lead to an acid digestive tract
10. cause premature aging

It is helpful to look at our relationship with sugar from an evolutionary perspective. We go crazy for the taste of sugar. In a natural hunter-gatherer's environment, it was rare to encounter many sweet foods. When they were available, it was generally for one season out of the year when fruits ripened. This is sugar contained within a natural matrix of fiber and essential micronutrients. From a survival perspective, it was beneficial to stop everything and gorge on ripe fruit when it was found. Fruit generally ripens one season prior to winter, and some extra fat reserves would be helpful. Of course, insulin levels would go up along with body fat, but since this was a once a year occurrence, it was no problem. This is all part of the metabolic cycling we will discuss later.

Compare this to the constant sugar availability and surplus we encounter today. While shopping at my local supermarket last week, the first thing I noticed while pulling into the store's parking lot were billboard advertisements for candy bars. I had not even made it out of my car and the messages were bombarding me. Enter the store and the first stack of food in front of you is usually a sugar-containing snack food. The candies and sodas occupy the end caps of the aisles, prime position for marketing. Going to a supermarket and not purchasing sugar-containing foods can be tough sometimes. Am I crazy or being a fanatic? Look at what everybody else is eating.

Some good news regarding sugar consumption is that our bodies and senses have a remarkable ability to auto-adjust our sensitivity to sweet. This means that after cutting out all added sugars, eliminating store-bought juices, cutting way back on dried fruits, and moderating fruit intake, a wonderful thing will happen. You will begin to taste sweetness in things that you never before realized were sweet.

After cutting my sugar intake, I was amazed to find that a raw red pepper really was sweet. With a few weeks of eating no sugar behind you, processed high-sugar foods will begin to feel distorted and unnatural. Eating sugar really is an addiction, and if you eat a typical Western diet you cannot imagine how addictive and pervasive sugar is until you are free of it.

Grains and the Carbohydrate Connection

This segment is interesting to write, as it goes against everything that I believed about nutrition and eating for many years. You may question its validity. But please keep an open mind. Remember, what stands in the way of enlightenment is not the things that we don't know, but the things that we think to be true that just are not so.

The incidence of obesity and diabetes is already at alarming rates in Western countries, and rapidly increasing around the world as the Western diet is adopted. Scientists are finally questioning the dogma of the last thirty years, which was the belief that dietary fat is the primary cause of obesity and metabolic diseases such as diabetes and heart disease. In the USA, through national nutritional policy, the average percentage of fat reduction in the diet went down from about 40% to 30% over the last thirty years, yet the incidence of obesity and metabolic diseases continues to climb. As Dr. Lustig points out in his videos on sugar and obesity, food manufacturers created new "low fat" versions of their products by reducing fat and adding sugar.

In all instances around the world where a Western diet consisting of a high concentration of refined grains and sugars is introduced to people who had formerly been eating an ancestral diet,

health rapidly declines and degenerative diseases become prevalent.[29] In his research article, "Comparison with ancestral diets suggest dense acellular carbohydrates promote an inflammatory microbiota, and may be the primary dietary cause of leptin resistance and obesity," Ian Spreadbury observes that all healthy ancestral diets share in common a complete absence of foods with a high-carbohydrate density.

Carbohydrate density is defined as the number of grams of carbohydrate contained in 100 grams of a food. For example, a pretzel has a carbohydrate density of 80. Rye crispbread is around 65. However, a carrot is around 8 and a sweet potato is about 15. Carbohydrate foods consumed in ancestral diets typically have very low carbohydrate densities and the carbohydrates are stored within the fiber walls. The low-density carbohydrates are locked in until the cell walls are broken in the digestive process and the carbohydrates are slowly absorbed. This slow absorption helps to prevent rapid changes in blood sugar and attendant spikes in insulin.

By contrast, the refined grains and sugars eaten in a Western diet have carbohydrate densities ranging from 65 to 100. Also, since these carbohydrates are acellular (broken down and separated from the plant cell) they digest very quickly, causing huge jumps in blood glucose and consequently spikes in insulin, then drops in blood sugar. Spreadbury observes in his research that when this high carbohydrate density food enters the GI tract, it enables the growth of a more inflammatory GI microbiota, which has a side effect of creating leptin resistance, hyperphagia (excessive hunger or increased appetite) and periodontal disease. Leptin is a powerful hormone made by fat cells that tells the brain whether to eat and store some more fat or to stop eating. In Western populations eating the diet of sugars, refined grains, and processed foods,

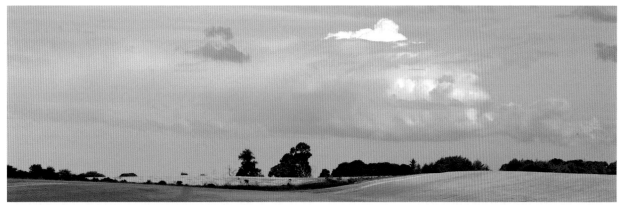

Scottish grain field — lovely to look at, but grains are good to avoid — especially those containing gluten, such as barley, wheat, and rye.

leptin resistance develops and leptin levels are far greater than in those eating a more ancestral diet with cellular, low-density carbohydrates.

Why Avoid Grains

There are other good reasons for avoiding grains and eating a lower carbohydrate diet. Grains contain many compounds that are classified as "anti-nutrients" and create havoc with our digestion and health.

Most grains contain phytic acid, which binds to minerals such as zinc, magnesium, iron and calcium, creating mineral deficiency. Interestingly, only ruminant animals possess the enzyme to break down phytic acid. That would seem to indicate that ruminants are meant to eat grains and not us humans. Phytic acid can be deactivated by fermentation, but it takes extremely long fermentation periods, on the order of 3 days. Very few of us make our own sourdough bread and ferment grains for that long.

Grains contain many compounds that are classified as "anti-nutrients" and create havoc with our digestion and health.

Grains also contain enzyme inhibitors. These are compounds that protect the seed from sprouting before the proper moisture conditions exist. They make digestion difficult. Enzyme inhibitors can be removed by soaking. However, the vast majority of grain consumed today is not soaked first.

Gluten is a well know problem with grains, and many people are allergic to this protein. Gluten can break down into lectin. It is found in most grains, although gluten-free products are now more available.

Lectins are well-studied proteins, and are responsible for some significant health issues when consuming grain. They are thought to play a role in plant's defences against being eaten. They play this role on a molecular level by binding to sugar structures of animal, fungal or microbial origin. Cooking or digestion does not break down lectins, and once inside us they have destructive effects. The minor ones are anti-nutritional and create allergic effects. However, as described in the research article, *Agrarian diet and diseases of affluence — do evolutionary novel dietary lectins cause leptin resistance?*[30], lectins are capable of binding to the insulin and leptin receptors, contributing to "diseases of affluence". These "diseases of affluence" include obesity, cardiovascular disease and diabetes.

The message is clear. Humans did not evolve eating grasses. We cannot break down the anti-nutrients in them and we need every advantage we can get to keep our insulin and leptin systems functioning properly in the toxic environment of our modern world. Try cutting grains out of your diet and see how you feel.

From Low Fat to Low Carb

For years I was a high-carbohydrate/low-fat eater and believed the best measure of dietary health was a curtailed fat content. I was able to tolerate this diet with a large intake of micronutrients from greens and other vegetables, but I often felt grouchy. But, eating high carb/low fat had become part of my personal dogma, much as it has become the official USDA food pyramid policy. Fortunately, I was willing to experiment with my diet, and in the process have found that a low-carb diet really changes the way that I feel in my body.

Here are some of the advantages of eating a low-carbohydrate diet:

- ◆ When you adapt to low carb and your body is burning fats instead of glucose, then the sensation of hunger changes. It becomes possible to just notice that you are hungry, instead of going crazy from low blood sugar and hunger urgency. Hunger will cease to control your life.

- ◆ In humans, low-carbohydrate diets reduce weight in a way that low-fat diets do not.[31] Low carbohydrate diets are prescribed in the treatment of diabetes and metabolic disease. But since all of us that have been eating western foods are pre-diabetic to one degree or another, we can benefit from the low-carb effect of reduced insulin resistance.[32]

- ◆ Paradoxically, eating a low-carb/high-fat diet improves cholesterol and blood lipid measures of cardiovascular disease.[33]

- ◆ You can finally eat some of the foods that were forbidden on a low-fat diet. In fact, when you eat a low-carb diet, the body preferentially burns saturated fats.[34]

- ◆ Better gut health and improved GI microbiota. Better regularity. This leads to fewer toxins in the body and improved mental acuity.

Try It and Feel Better

Go ahead. Try eating this way for 21 days and see how much better you feel. Probably the biggest challenge will be: "What do I eat once I remove grains and sugar?" Check out the recipes in Chapter 5 to start your exciting transformation.

Withdrawing from Carbohydrate and Sugar Addiction

How do you know if you are addicted? Without a sweet treat do you feel light-headed, tired or confused? Do the shakes or weakness get relieved shortly after eating something sweet? When you stop eating sugar do you get headaches, nausea or even vomiting? Do you swim up a river named "de-Nile" (denial)!

Anything you must have in order to avoid a negative feeling or symptom that tends to weaken the body as a result (even if you feel temporarily better) is an addiction.

We can become addicted both psychologically and physically. We can use food as a means to comfort ourselves beginning early on when we cry out for another bottle. Boredom, unhealed emotional hurts, unfulfilling work or relationships can all trigger feelings that scream out for soothing. Food, and especially carbohydrates, can distract us through the pleasure associated with the taste as well as numb us in our thinking and obsession with unresolved feelings.

Physically, eventually food is broken down in the digestive system and the liver and becomes glucose. The need to eat simple sugars, honey or fruit juices on a regular basis suggests an inability to break down complex foods into sugars. Thus a craving develops to reflect this inability, producing a desire to eat the end product — sugar. This creates a malfunction in the body and further clogs up the proper body signals.

There are many triggers in the body that work synergistically for and against our health. Even if we are careful about diet, if our adrenal gland activity is low, blood sugar levels will tend to be chronically low. To support adrenal health we need rich sources of vitamin C, E and B complexes as well as bioavailable copper, manganese, zinc, chromium, selenium, silicon and iron. If one is all vegan they can easily come up short in the vitamin B department and further the cycle of weakened adrenals. Improper absorption or lack of the proper vitamins and minerals is a huge component

of the many factors that can cause physical sugar addiction. Chronic stress and improper food nourishment (which is another form of stress on the body) can create a vicious cycle, further depleting the adrenals, causing a downward spiral.

How to Come Down From and Off Sugar Addiction

As you let go of carbohydrates and sugar, you will be coming down from a false high. Realize you will go through withdrawals. You might feel tired, dazed, confused, cranky, emotional, vulnerable, shaky, have a headache or flu-like symptoms. This too shall pass. Think of this as a sugar-detox. Follow these steps, one step at a time, leading you off of sugar.

- Avoid all sugar in your diet. Fruit must be reduced as in most cases it is mainly sugar and water. To help transition eat only berries, grapefruits, green apples, and apricots.
- Use superfoods such as barley grass and spirulina to give your body vital nutrients.
- Take a walk every day.
- Identify habits that feed the sugar habit. Notice when and why you want sugar.
- Until the problem is corrected eat smaller snacks more frequently to keep your blood sugar constant, helping to curb sweet cravings.

The Importance of Metabolic Cycling and the Benefits of Intermittent Fasting

Everything in nature occurs in cycles. Night turns to day. The moon waxes and wanes. Tides go in and out. Seasons roll from spring to summer, fall then winter. Rivers flood and dry up. There are long cycles and short cycles, and they are all combined on top of each other to create even more complex cycles such as weather patterns.

Our bodies evolved in this natural world, and were constantly subject to such cycles. As a result, the key cycles that affected the development of our human bodies were the cycles of feast and famine and exercise and rest. Our ancestors in the Paleolithic period did not have constant food availability as we do today. They lived in conditions where they would feast after a successful hunt or in seasons when fruit was abundant. Interspersed with the feasts were periods of famine from severe winter, summer drought conditions or unsuccessful hunts. Survival depended on the ability to store calories from feast periods and being able to turn these stored calories into energy during times of famine.

Contrast these conditions to our modern world. We live in a time of round-the-clock food availability. As noted previously, the number of eating occasions in the USA has climbed noticeably in recent years. Three meals a day is only the beginning, and for many, having five or six meals a day is standard practice. How many people do you know who regularly go a day or two without eating? Have you ever gone for a week without food? Unless we are in a war zone or something extreme, famine is just not part of our modern western world.

Combined with constant food availability is the change in physical lifestyle. None of us runs for miles and chases animals with a spear while starving and in freezing weather. Instead, we drive the car to the fast food drive-through or take something out of the freezer and pop it into the microwave and eat it on the couch while playing a video game. We live a life of sedentary ease and non-stop food abundance. Grok the caveman would be jealous.

Metabolic researchers believe that these changes of constant food availability and lack of intense physical activity have stalled an important metabolic cycle in our bodies, and this causes the range of metabolic diseases (obesity, insulin resistance, NAFLD, diabetes, hypertension, cancer, Alzheimer's, etc.) seen today.[35] As Chakravarthy and Booth note in their research, ancient man was genetically selected to have a "thrifty gene" from the constant cycling of fuel stores, blood insulin, insulin sensitivity and metabolic proteins driven by the constant cycles of feast-famine and physical activity-rest. So, our bodies evolved to have a natural metabolic state that required the constant cycling of the storage levels of glycogen and triglycerides, which was driven by the feast-famine and physical activity-rest cycles. This is what keeps us healthy. It's like the other cycles of nature. Things wouldn't work so well if the seasons got stuck in summer or winter.

What happens instead to our bodies in modern Western societies with continuous food abundance and sedentary lifestyles? We eat, rest and store fuel without the stimulus for utilizing it. Our bodies are very efficient at storing fuel, especially in the calorie-dense environment we have created for ourselves. But we rarely if ever go through the cycle of drawing down our energy stores of glycogen and triglycerides through the stimulus of famine or intense physical activity.

Our bodies do not receive the regular benefits of this required metabolic cycling that our system is designed to experience, and instead the cycle stalls with continuous high levels of glycogen and triglycerides stored in our muscles and liver. As a consequence we tend to develop the chronic metabolic diseases noted above. Intermittent fasting is a way to help create this natural metabolic cycle in our bodies. Please remember that in conjunction with intermittent fasting, regular physical exercise is also required to obtain the full benefits.

How Intermittent Fasting and Metabolic Cycling Feels in Your Body

Probably the most impressive part of the PURE 5:2 Transformation is the feeling in your body and your mental and emotional state when you start to experience repeated metabolic cycling. This is what happens when your body is allowed to burn fat. If you have been eating a pure high nutrient density diet, then your body has the essential phytonutrients, antioxidants, and enzymes that it needs to run properly and easily handle the cycles. It's like accelerating in your car when it's perfectly tuned.

Things really change when you fast long enough to burn up the glycogen stores in your muscles and liver. Your body has approximately 900 calories worth. After this point your body can enter a state called ketosis. During ketosis your brain and body is fuelled differently by burning fat rather than just burning glucose as you normally do. This is just one of the metabolic cycling benefits. What happens when you do an intense workout in the fasted state? Let me tell you from personal experience, it is a feeling unlike any other. Also, research has proven that working out in a fasted state can lead to efficient fat burning and more rapid weight loss. Don't even think about drinking that sugar-sweetened "athletic" drink before working out!

This is what the PURE 5:2 Transformation is all about. Twice a week you get to experience a complete metabolic cycle in your body. Everybody has different needs and tolerances regarding the proper frequency and depth of the cycle. But, the key point is this: by going through the metabolic cycle you get to experience a transformation. You will experience autophagy as the cellular debris is cleansed from your body. You will experience the cycle of consuming stored glycogen and triglycerides. After that, if you have been eating a low-carbohydrate diet, you will burn off all of your glycogen reserves and will enter ketosis. In ketosis, your body actually runs more efficiently and makes more energy per oxygen molecule used. It alters brain function, and ketosis is used as a natural therapy for certain neurological conditions such as epilepsy. Once your body has developed metabolic flexibility and adjusted to burning fat and entering ketosis, you will probably experience far sharper and crisper mental clarity than you have ever experienced before. Indeed, fasting has always been associated with increased spiritual clarity.

Our Ancestors, The Hunter-Gatherers

Think about the evolutionary natural selection scenario. Better yet, imagine that you are the caveman or cavewoman who has not eaten for days. It is the end of winter and your tribe has run out of food. The snowfall finally stops and now the hunt begins. You head out with 3 other villagers, on foot, armed with arrows and spears, to track and kill food for the starving tribe. Imagine your body at that point. No food for days. Freezing cold. Shivering hard to stay warm. (No warm car and drive-thru coffee and Egg McMuffin to start the day.) These are feelings that we don't have too often in modern times. You head out with your tribal family who are all just as cold and hungry as you are. As you cross a frozen lake to get to the best hunting ground, your party is ambushed by a pack of six hungry wolves. Big ones. At this point you are all sprinting towards the tree line at the edge of the frozen lake to get to the trees before the wolves get to you. Let me ask you a question: How alert and alive will you be feeling in your body? Will you have the energy that you need or will you complain about no breakfast and say you need an energy bar before a workout?

If you didn't have the mental acuity to be crisp and alert, and the burst of energy to outrun the wolves, then you were probably eaten. Over eons, the people who didn't were definitely the ones who were eaten, or just were unable to feed themselves and didn't pass on their genes. What that means is that the bodies that we are blessed with today are the ones that were selected to endure metabolic cycling and survive in feast/famine conditions and produce extreme physical output when needed. Which was often. That means you, too, can have an intense workout in the fasted state and have physical energy and mental clarity as you have never experienced before. This is the state that your body is genetically programmed to be able to enter. Outthink and outrun the wolves. Until you have experienced this you can't imagine how it feels. But it's real, and since this genetic programming lies latent within you, it means that you, too, can experience feeling this way. Perhaps you can try it twice a week?

Of course, you outran the wolves and dispatched a few of them with arrows once you climbed the trees. After that, you successfully hunted and killed a mastodon, then trekked 10 miles back to the village to summon help to cut up and retrieve this 4-ton prize.

Now ask your caveman self a question. Did you eat a lot over the next few days? Did you worry about your waist size going up an inch, or feel guilty if you missed a few workouts? Imagine how it must have felt in your body to go from starving and exhausted from the hunt, to relaxing around the fire gorging on freshly roasted mastodon brain

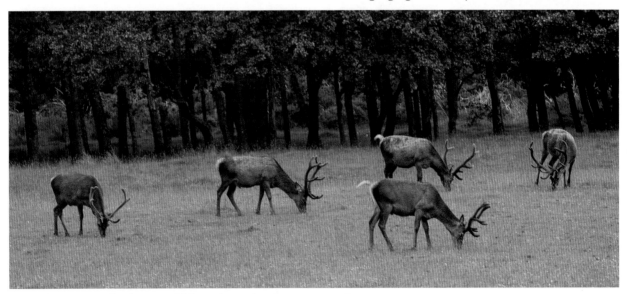

Wild deer — a sight that would have been familiar to our Paleo ancestors.

and liver. Yes, you would eat the prized, highest fat, most nutrient-dense organs first. Then, you would eat and eat, until you could eat no more. The next few days you would probably continue to feast and probably gain 10 pounds. It would feel wonderful to gain the weight because the stored energy meant survival and the ability to reproduce.

This is how our ancestors lived and experienced metabolic cycling. Only 500 generations ago, this is how humans were naturally selected and these selection pressures are what created the bodies that we have today. "A better understanding of many modern health problems will emerge when we consider that most of human evolution took place when our ancestors were hunter-gatherers."[36]

Scientifically Proven Health Benefits of Intermittent Fasting

Fasting has been a basic part of health and wellness practices in many different cultures throughout the recorded history of mankind.[37] This timeless tradition may be partially rooted in cellular and biochemical processes we are now beginning to understand in modern scientific terms. Intermittent fasting has been the subject of numerous controlled scientific studies and has been shown to have many different benefits. Here are some of the documented health benefits that you can expect from intermittent fasting.

Weight loss is one of the most obvious and desired benefits of intermittent fasting. In a 2009 study at

the Department of Kinesiology and Nutrition at the University of Illinois, 16 obese test subjects were put on an intermittent fasting weight loss program.[38] On the fast days their food intake was restricted to 25% of normal, and on the non-fast days they were allowed to eat all they wanted. This protocol did differ from the 5:2 program since every other day was a fast. So, if you are really interested in more rapid weight loss you could increase the number of fast days to match this study. The weight loss trial lasted for 8 weeks, after a 2-week control period. During this time, the subjects lost an average of over 12 pounds each. For half of the period the subjects were able to self select their food intake. Their weight loss during this period was the same as it was when the researchers controlled their food. This indicates that intermittent fasting is a diet program that is easy to follow.

In addition to losing weight, the test subjects also had significant improvements in their cardiovascular health measurements. Their total cholesterol, LDL cholesterol and triaclglycerol concentrations decreased by 21, 25 and 32% on average. Also, their systolic blood pressure decreased by 8mm Hg. on average.

Another study at the same lab compared weight loss with a constant calorie restriction diet versus weight loss through intermittent fasting.[39] They found that both programs yielded the same total weight loss, however, with intermittent fasting the test subjects lost less fat-free lean mass (muscle) than

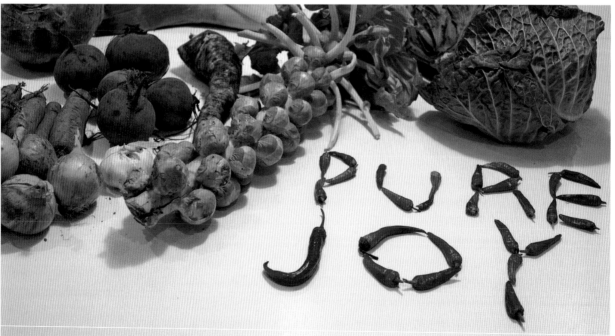

Our Christmas present from Jacqui of Strathconan.

Photo by Geoff Randolph

the subjects on a constant calorie restriction. This is a key finding, which verifies that intermittent fasting is a healthier way to lose weight.

In a wide range of species, the only environmental variable that has been shown to significantly affect the rate of aging is caloric intake. Reducing food to a level typically 30 to 40% less than that which would normally be consumed voluntarily results in a slowdown in the rate of aging and increase in maximum lifespan. This caloric restriction has also been shown to reduce kidney disease, cancer formation, and lessen neuron degeneration that is typical of Alzheimer's and Parkinson's disease. This is good news, but in practice it is extremely difficult to live a normal life on 60–70% of the food that you would normally eat. Very few people are really willing to endure such a regime long term!

However, researchers from the National Institute of Aging have found that when lab mice are fed an intermittent fasting diet regime with no restriction in total calories (which allows the mice to retain their normal weight), this resulted in the same benefits as a caloric restriction regime on their glucose and insulin levels and neuron resistance to excitotoxic stress.[40,41] In addition, researchers at UC Berkeley have shown that intermittent fasting reduces cancer risk and cell proliferation rates in mice as much as calorie restriction does.[42] These studies all indicate that intermittent fasting can provide the same health benefits as calorie restriction without the long-term drawbacks of eating 30-40% less food.

Enough talk about mice! What about research on humans? One of the key markers of metabolic health is insulin sensitivity. When diabetes develops, the body becomes less and less sensitive to insulin, and the pancreas must produce it in ever increasing quantities. Eventually, the pancreas fails to produce the insulin needed. So, the results of a study on healthy human subjects at the University of Copenhagen give hope for the usefulness of intermittent fasting in preventing the onset of diabetes.[43] In this study, eight healthy young men were put on an intermittent fasting regime for two weeks. During the feeding portion they ate enough so that their weight remained constant. This study showed that intermittent fasting increased the insulin sensitivity of the whole body. They concluded that cycles of feast and famine are important as an initiator of "thrifty genes" leading to improvements in metabolic function.

One cellular response to fasting is the activation of autophagy (from the Greek, "auto" oneself, "phagy" to eat). This is a process in which the cell self-digests its own components. This self-digestion not only provides vital nutrients to cells during fasting but also allows cells to rid themselves of undesirable components such as invading microorganisms, malformed or worn out proteins or damaged organelles (sub-structures within a cell). This self-cannibalistic process of autophagy keeps cells from becoming choked with trash and malfunctioning. It is triggered by fasting, exercise and certain dietary compounds and is now being seen as a biological pathway that functions to promote health and longevity. Proper autophagy is believed to help protect against a range of diseases, including infections, neurodegeneration, cancer, heart disease and aging.

There have been many more studies. Intermittent fasting has also been shown to reduce inflammation in asthma patients and reduce the risk of coronary artery disease. In addition, it is a way to boost the level of human growth hormone (HGH), which typically declines as we age. You can see the pattern here: intermittent fasting has been scientifically proven to work. All of these disease prevention benefits are wonderful, but what is really exciting about intermittent fasting is the way you can feel right now in your body when you put it into practice!

In summary, current research has shown these important and often unknown highlighted benefits of intermittent fasting:

◆ Normalizing insulin sensitivity, which is critical for optimal health as insulin resistance is a primary contributing factor to nearly all chronic disease, from diabetes to heart disease and even cancer

◆ Normalizing ghrelin levels, also known as "the hunger hormone"

◆ Promoting human growth hormone (HGH) production, which plays an important part in health, fitness and slowing the aging process

◆ Lowering triglyceride levels

Obesogens, or Why It's More Than Just Diet and Exercise

"There is nothing ulterior in our motives. Nothing at all. You will discover this for yourselves before too long. Simply by testing the various devices, which we will make available to you. We can show you for example, how to add a certain cheap fertilizer to the soil and end famine on Earth for good and all. We ask only that you trust us, only simply trust us."

Right. Guess how that episode of the *Twilight Zone* from the early 60s turned out. The poor Earthling on the loading dock of the "friendly alien space ship" learns all too late that the alien's book *To Serve Man* is actually a cookbook! This episode was at the same time that Monsanto built their ride in Disneyland's Tomorrow Land, which made us kids think that their vision for our future was magical and good. We could trust them, too.

What is going on in the world today is unprecedented in the history of humanity. There is something happening to our bodies. And it's making us fat. The global population continues to soar, and in conjunction obesity rates are steadily rising. This is happening in developing countries as well as industrialized countries. It is almost as if the world is becoming one big feedlot for *Homo sapiens*.

For one country this is already the case. The United States allows things in its food supply and environment that are strictly banned in most other countries. Unlabeled GMO foods, toxic chemicals, synthetically derived foods and hormones are present in the food stream and contaminate the air, land and water. Unfortunately, American-style agriculture, diet and environmental contamination is being spread around the globe, and it is estimated by the World Economic Forum that within two decades over half of the entire world will be overweight!

Many in the medical and exercise physiology world remain stuck in the idea that bad diet and lack of exercise are the only causes for obesity. While diet and exercise are certainly key factors, researchers have gathered convincing evidence that chemical obesogens are also major factors in the global rise of obesity. Obesogens are endocrine-disrupting chemicals found in our food and environment. They include pesticides, plastic-based and other industrial compounds, pharmaceuticals, growth hormones fed to animals and naturally occurring chemicals found in foods such as soy products. Since they disrupt the sensitive balance of the body's endocrine system, obesogens can cause unnatural weight gains.

Different obesogens cause weight gain in different ways. Some obesogens affect the size of fat cells. Other obesogens increase the number of fat cells, and there are others that affect hormones such

What is going on in the world today is unprecedented in the history of humanity. There is something happening to our bodies and it's making us fat.

as leptin that control food preferences, energy metabolism, and appetite. Obesogens can be so potent that they may pass on these changes to future generations through modifications to DNA.[44]

When I first read about obesogens, it all seemed a bit far-fetched. If we believe that obesity is caused by exposure to these obesogens in the environment, as well as changes in diet and activity levels, then how do you really test or determine if this is true or not? After all, the countries that have the greatest amounts of these chemicals in the environment are the same places where populations have adopted unhealthy western eating patterns and sedentary lifestyles. How do you independently show that something is really happening on account of the obesogens?

Fortunately for our understanding of the effects of obesogens, we humans are not the only the only living creatures affected by this increase of obesogens in the environment. Scientists have confirmed that animals inhabiting human-influenced environments are also showing weight gain. In the research paper "Canaries in the coal mine: a cross-species analysis of the plurality of obesity epidemics,"[45] scientists examined samples collectively consisting of over 20,000 animals from 24 different populations and studied for an average of 15-year periods. The animals studied included both feral, domestic and lab animals, all in environments that were influenced by human activity. For all of the animal populations, the trend for weight over time was positive. They were all gaining weight and becoming more obese. The chance of this happening randomly is less than one in 12 million. This was in the absence of the reasons usually given for obesity in humans: changes in diet and activity.

Something is happening in our environment, and it is affecting the animals as well as us humans. What are these obesogens and where do we find them?

Obesogens are everywhere around us. They are in our food, water, shampoo and cosmetics, plastic bottles, cars, cookware, carpets, store receipts and even paper money. It is impossible to completely avoid exposure to them living on planet Earth these days. However, by understanding what they are, and where they are hidden, we have a fighting chance to avoid many of them and make it easier to lose weight and stay healthy. Here are the main categories of obesogens and where they are hidden:

◆ Hormones and antibiotics in meat and dairy

The industrial meat and dairy industries in the United States routinely add antibiotics to the feed and implant synthetic growth hormones into the animals to increase the weight gain or amount of milk produced per unit of feed. These hormones are powerful synthetic estrogens that leave residues. They can have the same effect on human bodies as they do on the animals. It is interesting to note that these practices are banned in Europe but are still allowed in the USA. American meat raised with hormones cannot be imported into Europe. The obesity rates in Europe are much lower than they are in the USA, and this could be one factor. As with hormones, antibiotics in animal feed are not allowed in Europe but they are allowed in the USA. These antibiotic residues may alter the delicate balance of the bacteria in our gut, which can affect how we metabolize our food.

◆ Pesticides and herbicides

Some of the major sources of persistent organic pollutants (POP) in our environment are agricultural pesticides, herbicides and fungicides. One of the first pesticides to be identified as highly dangerous was DDT, but it is still in use around the world today. Its breakdown product, DDE, is linked to insulin resistance in rodents and increased BMI (body mass index) in children.[46] Given the globalization of the food supply, if a pesticide is used anywhere on Earth, it means that you could be unknowingly eating it!

Another common herbicide in use today with strong obesogenic properties is Atrazine. This dangerous chemical is used primarily on cornfields in the USA, and its use has been dramatically increasing recently as glyphosate herbicides have lost their effectiveness against superweeds. A Korean study in 2009 showed that even low levels of Atrazine in animals drinking water had the effects of decreased basal metabolic rate, increased body weight, increased intra-abdominal fat and increased insulin resistance without changing the food intake or physical activity level.[47] The researchers also note that Atrazine is routinely found as a contaminant in the surface and ground waters where it is applied. It is disturbing to note that the corn growing regions where Atrazine is most heavily used are also the regions of the USA with the most obesity. Coincidence?

Something to remember with food-borne obesogens is that they become concentrated in animal products. A steer may eat 10 pounds of grain to produce 1 pound of meat. The organic pollutants in the feed tend to get concentrated in the fat cells of animals. The grains raised for animal feeds are usually GMO herbicide tolerant varieties and are heavily sprayed with herbicides.

Due to the dangers of Atrazine, it has been banned in Europe. However, as with many other dangerous chemicals that have been banned in Europe, it is still allowed in the USA.

◆ Flame retardants, non-stick compounds and plasticizers

Flame retardants, non-stick compounds and plasticizers are potent endocrine disrupting obesogens that are ubiquitous in our modern lives. The flame retardant PBDE and non-stick compound PFOA (perfluorooctanoate) are found nearly everywhere: in carpets, waterproof clothes, furniture, non-stick cookware, mattresses and packaging of microwaveable foods. Virtually everyone in industrialized countries has detectable levels of these compounds in their blood, and they can have damaging effects on the next generation. For example, in a recent journal article, researchers studied 665 Danish women who were pregnant in the late 1980s and the levels of PFOA were measured in their blood.[48] The researchers analyzed BMI of their offspring 20 years later in 2009. They found daughters of women who had about 6 parts per billion of PFOA in their serum had an average BMI 1.6 greater compared to daughters of women who had about 2 PPB of the PFOA in their blood. The male offspring were unaffected.

The plasticizer BPA (Bisphenol A) is one obesogen that has received much public attention lately. This chemical is used in food can liners, store receipts, polycarbonate bottles and dental sealants. In the USA alone, industry consumes over 2 billion pounds of BPA per year. However, its use in baby bottles has been banned in the USA and Europe. BPA reduces the number of fat cells, but causes them to be much larger, thus creating more fat.

Phthalates are a type of plasticizer used in PVC plastics, plastic films, and also in scented products such as laundry items, air fresheners, cosmetics, shampoos, and soaps. More than 75% of Americans have measurable levels of phthalates in their urine. Phthalates reduce testosterone levels in men, and studies have shown a positive correlation between phthalates concentration in urine and the waist circumference and insulin resistance in US men.[49]

◆ **Pharmaceuticals and food**

Many of the commonly used pharmaceuticals today have obesogenic effects. Prescription antidepressants, diabetes drugs and DES synthetic estrogen have all been shown to be obesogenic. The modern trend to overprescribe antibiotics means that the average child in the USA has received 10–20 courses of antibiotics by the time that they are 18 years old. This is significant because our guts contain over 1,000 different species of microorganisms that help to regulate our metabolism. Altering this balance with antibiotics can affect fat storage.[50]

Certain food items also act as obesogens. For example, the use of soy-based infant formula that contains the estrogenic component genistein has been associated with obesity later in life.[51] Probably the most prevalent obesogen in our modern food is MSG (mono-sodium glutamate). MSG consumption has been shown to correlate with increased body mass index.[52] MSG is hidden in most processed foods using dozens of innocent sounding names, so it is easy to unknowingly consume this obesogen if you eat processed foods or are eating out.[53]

Avoiding Obesogens

So, now that you know about obesogens, what do you do? They are in our homes, workplaces and everywhere in our environment, so they are impossible to totally avoid. But, with some awareness and basic actions, you can avoid exposure to most of them. Here is a list of actions you can start today:

◆ Buy organic foods, preferably unpackaged and from farmers at local markets. Organic is especially important for animal products and fat-containing foods, as toxins bio-accumulate in animal tissues and tend to be fat-soluble.

◆ Avoid farm-raised fish and choose wild-caught whenever possible.

◆ Avoid processed, pre-packaged foods, especially canned, whenever possible.

◆ Get a good quality water filter.

◆ Minimize plastics whenever possible in your life. Avoid having plastics touching your food

or water, and never ever cook or microwave food in plastic containers. If you must microwave foods, take it out of the plastic container first.

◆ Avoid microwaved popcorn.

◆ Be sure that your cosmetics, personal care products and fragrances come from natural sources.

◆ Specifically avoid products with parabens or phthalates.

◆ Avoid handling cash register receipts. If your job involves touching them all day then wear gloves.

◆ Use chemical-free cleaning products and avoid anti-microbial soaps and toothpastes.

◆ Don't drink water that has been sitting in a garden hose.

◆ Get rid of all non-stick cookware. Once you use a good cast iron pan you will be hooked. Also, it will never wear out, unlike Teflon.

◆ Avoid eating soy products and foods containing added MSG. Please note that manufacturers hide added MSG by using other names such as yeast extract, hydrolyzed protein, calcium caseinate, textured protein and others.

This is a lot to remember and do, but the results are worth it. Obesogens may be affecting your weight, growth, sexual function, sleep, mood, reproduction, stress and allergies. Whatever you can do to reduce your exposure to these dangerous chemicals will only add to the benefits of the PURE 5:2 transformation.

Focus on a Healthy Lifestyle, Not Weight Loss

I grew up with plenty of role models on how to count calories and Weight Watcher points. I counted both to fall asleep at night! All the calorie counting never taught me a thing about eating foods to build up my immune system, not tear it down. Sure, I could lose weight eating the prepackaged and pre-weighed foods but inevitably my cravings would come back and so would my low energy, compromised immune system and the ever-familiar cycle of guilt, binge, crash. Big business weight-loss companies can teach you to lower calories by switching to using "diet" drinks or chemical sweeteners. They don't teach you how using these products can create serious health issues. The key is to focus on living a healthy lifestyle, using wisdom through educating yourself about what is truly the best choice for your overall health.

Gut Feelings About Diet and Mental Health

The tenth cranial nerve that runs from the brain stem to the abdomen, known as the vagus nerve, is the main passageway by which gut bacteria travels to the brain. Dr. Natasha Campbell-McBride, a medical doctor based in London with a degree in neurology, asserts that toxicity from your gut can flow throughout the body into the brain where it can cause symptoms of autism, ADHA, depression, schizophrenia and other mental and behavioral disorders. She believes it is important for us to nourish and maintain good gut bacteria our whole lives. They say: "It all begins in the gut!"

Steps Towards a Healthy Gut and a Happy Mind!

- ◆ Avoid processed, refined foods
- ◆ Take a high-quality probiotic supplement
- ◆ Eat traditionally made, unpasteurized, fermented foods: The best thing is to eat traditionally made fermented raw foods (not pasteurized). These foods contain extremely beneficial "good" bacteria that help to reduce toxicity by being chelators of heavy metals and pesticides. Eating a variety of fermented food yields the widest spectrum of good bacteria as well as the added benefit of being a great source of vitamin K2. One serving of home-fermented food using the proper starter culture can contain 10 trillion beneficial bacteria as well as 500mcg of vitamin K2, a vital co-nutrient to vitamin D and calcium.

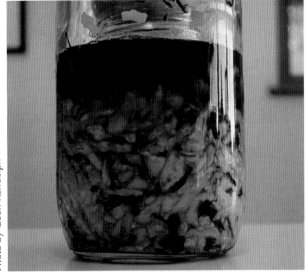

Photo by Geoff Randolph

Fermenting cabbage — using a heavy stone to press down the suaerkraut in process

Healthy fermented food choices include:

Fermented vegetables (we love red cabbage)

Lassi, an Indian yogurt drink

Kefir, which is fermented milk and comes in fruit flavors

Natto (fermented soy), which can be used in miso soups, sauces, and salad dressings

- ◆ Avoid antibiotics unless critical, and replenish your gut with probiotics and fermented foods afterwards. Eat all organic, grass-fed meats and animal products. Stay away from GMO, processed, and sugary foods. Avoid chlorinated and fluoridated water, antibacterial soap, and all agricultural chemicals.

- ◆ Stay away from glyphosate, a potent mineral chelator and active ingredient found in Monsanto's Roundup. When a plant has been exposed to glyphosate, minerals like zinc and magnesium get bound up and prevented from being used by the plant. Glyphosate gets integrated into plant cells, hence eating plants that have been exposed creates a binding of important minerals in the human body. Research indicates that zinc deficiency is a common factor in Alzheimer's and Parkinson's.

According to an article titled "How Agriculture Chemicals and Hospital Stays Contribute to Alzheimer's" by Dr. Mercola, avoiding gluten, getting plenty of the healthy fats (including butter, avocados, and coconut oil) and fasting all contribute significantly to proper brain health.

Glyphosate is patented as an antibiotic and, like all antibiotics, indiscriminately kills both beneficial and detrimental bacteria found in soil and the human gut. Mercola points out that glyphosate affects beneficial bacteria so that pathogens overgrow and take over. The body then has to deal with the toxins produced by the pathogens, leading to chronic inflammation, which is the root of chronic and debilitating disease.

"Old habits lose their grip, not by self-coercion, but by attraction to new habits sparking an awakened sense of aliveness." – David Sandoval

We have provided you with a 21-day plan so you can feel in your body what a difference it makes to eat PURE foods. Along with the suggested protocol, recipes and menu suggestions we recommend two essential elements that cannot be skipped if you want to experience PURE 5:2 Transformation in 21 Days. The first is some form of daily exercise. For the maximum results we suggest you learn about high intensity interval training (HIIT). At the very least we recommend 20–30 minutes of fast-paced walking. Whenever possible, add in some stretching or yoga.

Read on to find out about the second essential element to maximum success with PURE 5:2 Transformation in 21 Days.

NOTE: See references 54 through 63 on page 178 for articles cross-referenced in this chapter.

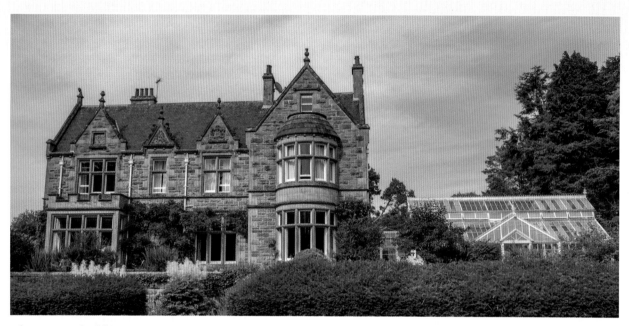

Above: Newbold House, community, retreat and workshop center in Forres, with its wonderful organic and sustainable gardens.

Below: The beach at Nairn on New Year's Eve.

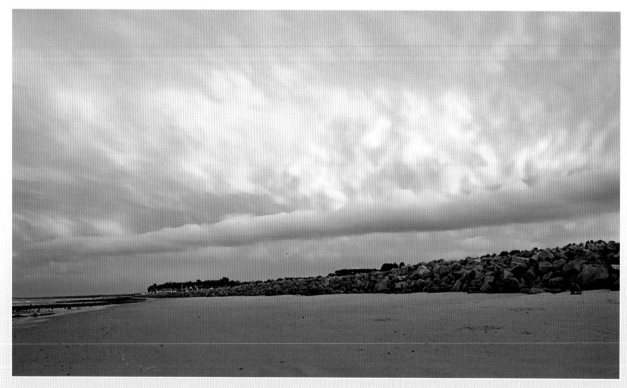

Photo by Robyn Randolph

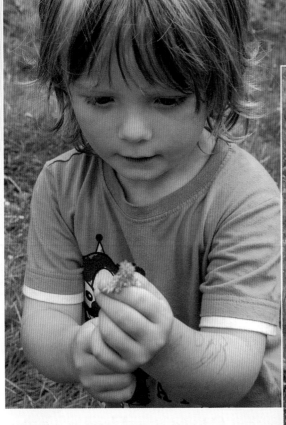

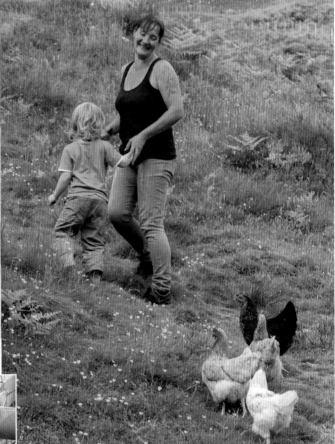

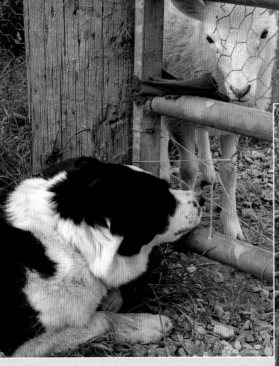

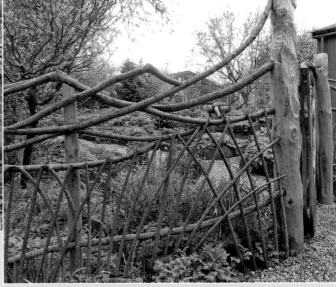

*Working in the original
world famous Findhorn Gardens*

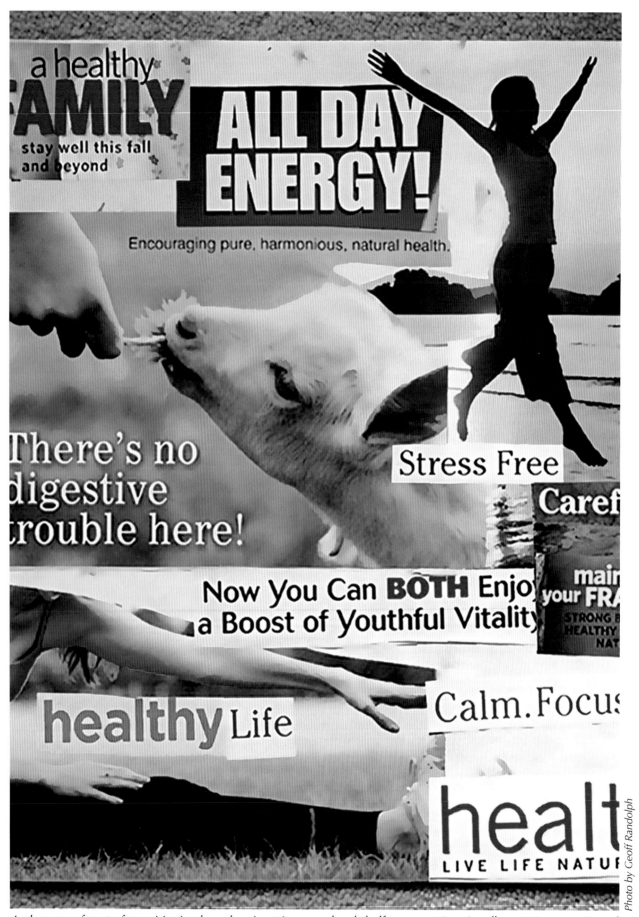

A close-up of part of my visioning board — I put it on my bookshelf so every time I walk past, I can see it and reinforce the direction I am heading.

CHAPTER 4
5:2 Days and Intuitive Eating

Don't Make Food Your Religion… Make It Your Wisdom!

How can any one diet be for all people? We are all unique. Different bodies require different things. If you are a sprouting teen, your body requirements are quite different from a woman plunging into menopause. Refining our diet is a process. Different foods and beliefs about eating seem to evolve as we evolve given our unique metabolisms and circumstances.

If you had told me 16 years ago that I would be happy eating lots of raw foods with some PURE, organic grass-fed animal products thrown in the mix I would have said … "no way"!

What matters is **what works well for you and what works well for you over time**. Stay flexible and keep checking in with yourself and track what brings more lightness, delight, energy, vitality, and sense of well-being.

In the times we live in, what matters NOW is how PURE is the food you are eating? This is crucial and foundational for the health of every one of us.

Learn as much as you can about food. Who are the healthiest people with the longest lives on this planet? What do our ancestors have to teach us about food? What is the current understanding about intermittent fasting?

Learn as much as you can, and then be still and **listen to your own body**. There are many dieting and health programs beckoning you to follow, PURE 5:2 included. We believe no one knows your body and your daily needs like you do. Experiment and find what works and what doesn't work, and let your intuition be wed with wisdom along the way.

What Is Intuitive Eating?

Whether you have health and/or weight loss goals in mind, the other essential ingredient for maximum results for PURE Transformation in 21 Days is Intuitive Eating. This is the key to unlock you from your "food issues" prison. It is the way you can lead yourself out of the danger zone…out of the pit of resistance and reactionary eating. It is the catalyst to go from reaction to mindful action and from there, to transformation.

A basic premise of Intuitive Eating is **on a gut level it should make sense!**

Intuitive Eating helps to connect you with the part of yourself that truly wants to nourish yourself. The wise you knows what you need to feed yourself in a way that promotes the very best for your health and well-being.

To help you get in touch with this part of you, here are some starting guidelines. Think of your "intuitive eating ability" much like your abilities to see, hear, taste, touch and smell. It is another amazing sense that you are capable of developing, just like you can develop any of your other senses.

The essence of this ability is about listening to the calm, wise, inner knowing that you can tap into by being present… not trying!

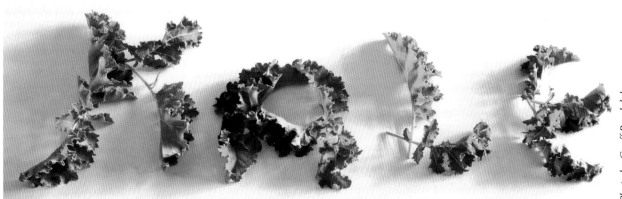

Photo by Geoff Randolph

K-A-L-E spells high nutrient density, PURE food!

Get yourself a special journal for your PURE Transformation in 21 Days and begin by answering the following questions.

Answer these questions from a place of non-attachment to outcome. Create a place inside your inner landscape where it is safe to just say what is true without judging yourself. Be authentic with yourself. Cultivate a gentle compassion and understanding for yourself, as if you were talking with a beautiful child who just wants to tell you what they notice about themselves and their behavior. How would you make it safe for that child to just be open and honest? Be that for yourself. Be the "witness to your process". Just observe as if you were in an anthropology class learning about this human being (who just happens to be you). Be a detached observer of yourself. Observe and report about the habits you discover about yourself. Take note of what you observe without any criticizing or judgmental words. Just report the facts. "I notice I eat chocolate when I feel lonely or stressed."

Please read each "coaching" question using your intuition (tapping into your inner knowing /wisdom and the part of you that desires to take the best care of yourself). Simply ask yourself the question, and then sit quietly and digest what you have read. Listen in the stillness (from a place of receptivity) until an answer bubbles up. Remember, there is no right or wrong. It just is what it is. Your role right now is communicating with yourself while also being the observer of yourself. The less you analyze the better.

Your intuition knows what is true, and that truth presents itself as a calm, gentle fact.

1. **What do you sense is the right balance for you?**

   Eating all raw, vegan? Eating mostly raw with some cooked vegan foods? Eating a balance of raw and cooked foods, including some fish? Eating animal products with raw foods? Or, perhaps some other type of combination...

2. **Do you eat when you are not hungry, and if so why do you think that is?**

3. **If so, is there a particular time you eat when you are not hungry?**

4. **Are you aware of any feelings present when you eat when you are not hungry?**

5. **Considering your current diet, are you satisfied when you eat?** If not, why do you think that is?

6. **What patterns do you have if any, around food?**

7. **What is your earliest memory of where those patterns began?**

8. **What did you learn about eating and food and your relationship with food from your family life?**

   ➤ For example: *"What I learned about food: I had to hurry up and eat fast; if I didn't, everyone else would be back for seconds, gobbling it up before I even got my first helping down. I also learned that going back for seconds, constant eating and thinking about food seemed 'normal.'"*

9. **Describe your relationship with food as if it were a relationship with a person.**

   ➤ For example: *"My relationship with food is on again, off again. I use food and food uses me!"* or *"I don't pay much attention to food..."* etc.

10. **Based on your answers, what do you know about yourself, and what works and what doesn't?**

    Feel free to write as much as you can about what you observe and know about yourself and your patterns. When you have taken as much time as you need to do this, turn the page.

11. **The consequences of what I observe with my relationship with food are...**

    On a fresh page, answer this question, writing as much as you can possibly think of.

Intuitive Visioning

Now that you see and know these things, let's focus on what you truly want.

1. **Turn the page.** This blank page is where you get to write how it is according to **how you want it to be.** Look at your fresh new page. It is a blank page. Your past is your past. You have a blank page and you are free to have a new relationship with food.

2. On this blank page, write about what that relationship with food looks like and speak as if **it already is.** Write in the present tense, in great detail about how you feel, what you do, what results you experience. Write everything from a positive perspective not mentioning anything from past behaviour. Don't talk about what you don't want… write about what you do want, as if it were already happening.

   ➤ For example: *"I love my relationship with food. I now know how to eat foods in a way where I feel completely satisfied. I use food to nourish my body and it is easy for me to make PURE 5:2 a lifestyle. In fact, I love doing 5:2 so much, it has become effortless."*

   "I naturally have balanced weight that is perfect for my unique body and metabolism. My weight has adjusted easily. I am free in a way I have never felt free in my relationship with eating/food."

   "I feel vibrant energy and am enjoying great health."

   Keep seeing and sensing what you would look, feel and be like now that you can write what it is you intuitively know it can be. Take your time and write as much as you possibly can.

3. **Turn the page.** Once you can see clearly what it is you want, write that in a condensed **Intuitive Intention Statement** using one or two sentences. Start out with these words:

   "I intend to create the possibility… and now write either *"to have"* or *"to be."*

   ➤ For example: *"I intend to create the possibility of being completely at peace with my relationship with food, eating a PURE 5:2 diet with ease and grace and feeling the most vibrant, healthy, and trim I have ever felt."*

4. **Write this Intuitive Intention Statement on several index cards,** and put them in places that remind you to stop and read those words. In your car you can read it at traffic lights. Put it by the sink (washbasin) to read when you brush your teeth or above the sink when you do dishes.

5. **Turn the page.**

   Title this page: **Step-by-Step Intuitive Intention Action Plan**

6. **On this page get quiet and listen.** Let your intuition direct you one step at a time as you answer the question below:

   What specifically are your next steps to take you towards fulfilling your intentions? (Once you accomplish the next step, what is the next step to take after that, and so on until you reach your intention.)

7. **As you approach each new day of the 21 days of PURE Transformation:**

   Re-read your:

   ◆ **Intuitive Visioning** – page or pages of seeing what you want in terms of your relationship with food, eating, your health, weight, etc.

   ◆ **Intuitive Intention Statement** – condensed statement written on index cards stating clearly the possibility you intend to create

   ◆ **Step-by-Step Intuitive Intention** – action plan on how to manifest your intention. Let your intuition and wisdom lead.

8. **Daily, as you approach food, let your intuition guide you to eat in a way that will take you where you want to go, always being sensitive to take the next best step towards your intention.**

If where you want to go is to lose unwanted pounds, then use your intuition when selecting food that day. Ask yourself before eating cookies if that is what will take you where you want to go!

Just ask your intuition, without counting calories, grams of fat or protein, if your food choices will help or hinder your weight and healthy lifestyle goals. Keep checking in with yourself. Keep that inner dialogue going and your relationship with food healthy, vibrant, and authentic.

Keep journaling and observing your choices.

Journaling, Intuitive Visioning, Intuitive Intention Statement and Daily Log (read further) are essential ingredients in nourishing you toward the optimal results for PURE Transformation in 21 Days.

Intuitive/Creative Weight Loss

The fact remains that most weight loss is a result of less calories in than calories burned. So on a "2 day", the less calories you consume the more chance of the math working out in your favour over the course of all the calories consumed and burned off for that 7 day period. However, as a culture, we have to lighten up on the whole counting calorie thing. For some people it creates obsessive behaviour. Who needs that? Raise your hand! Counting calories misses the mark in terms of quality of the calories consumed and how that synergistically affects your overall metabolism and health.

Quality, nutrient dense food that keeps our blood sugar stable is what we are truly after. Specifically, quality proteins and fats and restricting carbohydrates will yield you transformation. Stay the course on this for 21 days and you will experience PURE 5:2 Transformation in 21 Days!

Instead of worrying about every bite or calorie, just intuitively nourish yourself in a way that keeps in mind that the less calories the better, while fuelling yourself with low glycemic carbohydrates yet high nutrient density foods. Forget scales and tape measures. Your clothes don't lie. When you put the focus on eating for health, wellness and longevity the weight will adjust according to your overall metabolic balance. Keep your aim on eating PURE 5:2 and intuitively eating to nourish yourself.

During the course of the day keep listening to your body. If you begin to feel a bit hungry, see what beverage you could drink right then that would be most nourishing and in alignment with what it is you are wanting for your outcome that day. See how long you can go with just nourishing beverages and keep listening to what your body may need.

There have been some "2 days", depending on how active we might be that day, we both have found an intuitive inspiration to munch on raw food in the late afternoon. Geoff often will gravitate towards a couple leaves of fresh kale and graze as if he were a giraffe, while I like to eat a whole red bell pepper as if it were an apple.

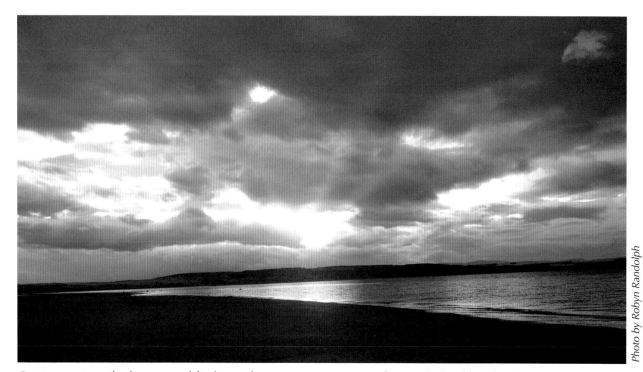

Getting out into the beauty and fresh air of nature is restorative and part of a healthy lifestyle.

Always do whatever you intuitively feel is the best thing for your body. Find what works for you. If a "2-day" isn't working out for you for some reason, you can always incorporate another "2 day" when you are more prepared. Just keep working with your own unique needs. Give yourself permission to be flexible around this whole 5:2 regime.

Stop and ask yourself these questions before you break your fast:

1. Do I need to eat for health/blood sugar reasons? If so, what would be the very best thing to nourish me right now?

2. What is the reason I want to break the fast now?

Be still and listen for the answer that is in alignment with what your healthiest goal is for yourself.

Keep imagining what it would look like and feel like to be healthy, well and a balanced eater with a good relationship with food. How would you look and act with food if you were taking the best care of yourself? How would you feel and be transformed from who you have always known yourself to be? What would you do differently? How do you see yourself choosing and preparing food?

Intuitively sense what you would be like with this new relationship with food. Describe that in full detail in you Intuitive Visioning journal writing. Feel free to keep adding to what you write and see if you can feel what it would feel like to live life in relationship with food this way.

Optional: Cut out pictures and paste on a vision board (poster board, thick paper, or cardboard). Incllude anything that is a visual cue of what it is you are imagining as your possibility. Be as creative as you want. Look at your poster board several times a day and feel the excitement connected to the visual cues. Create the possibility one step at a time to live what it is you are imagining and seeing represented by the pictures on your vision board.

Let these 21 days be filled with fun, creativity and the delight of going on a healthy transformation adventure.

I put my visioning board on my bookshelf so every time I walk past, I can see it and reinforce the direction I am heading! I used images that invoke specific meaning. The stack of stones, for example, represents my desire for balance. When I see the stones I affirm balance in my "inner visioning". I might even say to myself: "I am living a healthy, balanced life full of joy and energy!" The empty fork represents great "2 days."

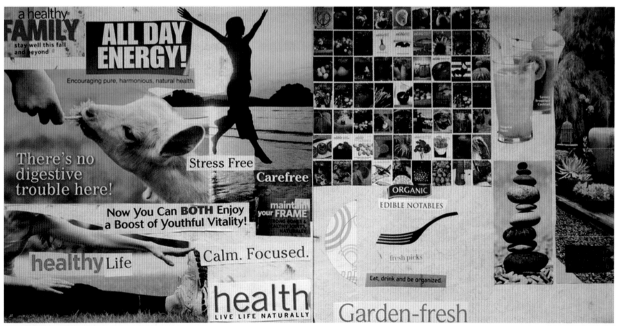

Find pictures and words to express your vision for how you want to "be" living a healthy lifestyle and paste them on a board.

Every day for the PURE Transformation in 21 Days please fill out the following daily log. This way at the end of the 21 days you can go back and track your progress. This will also help you know what works and what does not as you move forward. You can copy this page or make it a daily journal entry. Fill this out for every one of the 21 days.

Before each meal, please record: Day # _____

1. Time of Day

2. "Inner Awareness" **prior to eating**: record current hunger level vs. desire for food. Notice your thoughts, emotions, feelings and body sensations.

3. Ask yourself, "How hungry am I on a scale of 1–10?" 1 is "not at all," and 10 is "extremely."

Post-meal, please record:

4. Food or beverage eaten with detailed description. Quantity.

5. "Inner Awareness" after eating:
   Make notes about how you feel, satisfaction level, fullness, emotions, any thoughts or body sensations or possible triggers.

At the end of the day:

At the end of the day, do a quick review of your overall day and answer the following questions. (This process helps to make eating a more conscious experience).

1. On a 1–10 scale, 10 being fantastic, please rate the following:

   ◆ Energy level:

   ◆ Mental clarity:

   ◆ Feeling balanced (overall well-being):

   ◆ Blood sugar stability:

   ◆ Emotional balance (mood swings):

2. What liquids and how many ounces did you consume today?

3. Please comment on any noticeable symptoms or body responses.

4. Other than fruits and vegetables, what carbs did you have today?

5. Did you have any alcohol, sugar or caffeine?

6. How pleased are you with your choices and food intake amount today?

7. Did you consciously think about and practice "eating less food?"

8. In what ways did you practice Intuitive Eating?

9. Did you read your **Intuitive Vision Journaling** and **Intuitive Intention Statement** index cards?

How to Do the 21 Days
(Getting Organized)

1. **Read this entire book** so you get a clear overview of why and how you are doing this.

2. Break down the 21 days into 3 weekly segments, focusing on **one week at a time.**

3. Each week, **pick out recipes** we've suggested that intuitively attract you and map out which ones you want for **your "2 days"** and which ones you want for **your "5 days"** (or use your own choice of recipes on "5 days").

4. Put together a list of ingredients for that week. Try and do one big shop **the day before** you start your week so you are all organized. You may need to shop for fresh produce before the week is over. Always shop the day before the next week begins.

5. For best results we highly recommend you include spirulina and barley grass as much as possible, but not a deal breaker if you can't for some reason.

6. For these 21 days, eliminate all foods on the restricted food list (see list).

7. Create a special journal and follow steps outlined for Intuitive Eating and Visioning as well as filling out your daily log.

8. Get daily exercise.

9. Check our website: **purehighlandliving.com** for updates, blog posts, or new recipes.

Shopping list for each week:

"2 Days:"

◆ Homemade vitamin and mineral waters, teas, soups, broths, smoothie ingredients

◆ Fresh juices (**Option:** 10-Day Transformation pack ingredients. See details under **PURE "2 Days"** Transformation Easy Option.*)

◆ Mostly raw dinners to break the fast. Keep these dinners easy and simple.

◆ Can include soups or broths.

"5 Days:"

◆ Intuitively PURE breakfast and lunch

◆ Liquids throughout the day

◆ Intuitively PURE dinners

Restricted Foods List

◆ All packaged, processed foods

◆ All fats except butter, coconut oil, olive oil or Udo's choice

◆ All grains

◆ All forms of sugar except banana/dates/raisins (use very sparingly)

◆ All beans and legumes (use very sparingly)

◆ All alcohol

◆ All cow milk products

NOTE: If you have blood sugar issues use only stevia as a sweetener, and make sure to use one heaping tablespoon of coconut oil in juices and smoothies to keep your insulin from spiking. The key to success is keeping your blood sugar stable and as balanced as possible.

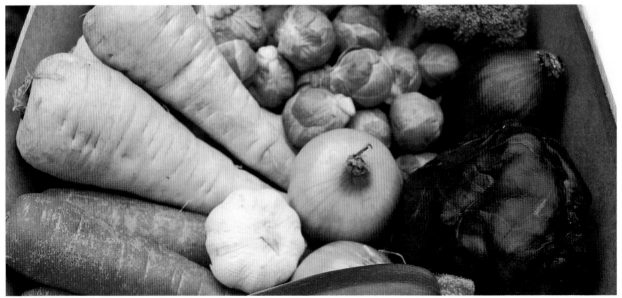

Photo by Robyn Randolph

Fresh veggie box from Strathconon Organix.

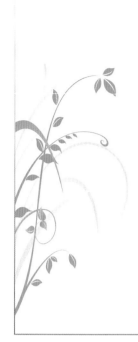

Summary of the Ideal Key Components of
PURE 5:2 Transformation in 21 Days

- Intermittent fasting (or modified intermittent fasting) so as to transform from burning carbs to burning fat as your primary metabolic fuel

- Eating lots of raw foods, including fermented foods and sprouts (particularly sunflower seed sprouts)

- Avoiding sugars, refined foods, processed foods, fruit juices as well as eliminating most fruit

- Shifting from poor-quality protein to high-quality protein

- Eating the right types of fats. Include one serving of MUFA (monounsaturated fatty acid) foods with every meal (see more MUFA information under PURE "5 Days" below)

- Eliminating all grains

- Drinking plenty of lemon water as well as barley grass three times a day

---

PURE "5 Days"

RawSome PURE is how we like to eat on our "5 days" (meaning mostly **RAW** with **SOME** cooked PURE food). A nice goal each week is to keep adding in **new, intuitively PURE recipes**; simple recipes or combinations of PURE foods that you create from what you sense would be nourishing to your body. Additionally, gradually shift over the balance of cooked to raw food to what you intuitively feel is best for your body. **Aim anywhere between 60–75% RAW to 25–40% SOME cooked ratio.**

One approach that works well is to mix raw foods with some cooked at every meal. This can be accomplished by dividing the plate into fourths (¾ raw, ¼ cooked) making it easy to see how much raw to put on the plate versus cooked.

Other people prefer to eat all raw until dinnertime, where some cooked food is added to a mostly raw meal. Each person has to find what works best to make a healthier eating lifestyle do-able and not something that is too extreme, confusing or too consuming.

Many people find that getting on a routine or regime is the key to success for a lifestyle change that results in dropping accumulated weight and toxins. Here are some helpful suggestions to incorporate into a daily action plan. Choose to take action, to manifest in physical form the changes you intuitively intend.

- Start your day by reading your **Intuitive Intention Statement**

- Upon arising, add the **juice of a fresh lemon** to 8–16 ounces of warm water. *Optional:* Add a teaspoon of Manuka honey and stir well. Wait half an hour before ingesting anything else. Drinking lemon water is a great way to flush out toxins and help your body to alkalinize. It also aids liver function.

- If time permits, drink another eight ounces of water mixed with one teaspoon of **barley grass powder.** Again wait for about 20 minutes before ingesting anything else.

- Drink another **green drink (barley or wheatgrass powder)** about a half hour prior to dinner. (One teaspoon of powder mixed in with eight ounces of water, carrot juice or coconut water, twice a day is a great goal). If you are new to powdered green drinks start with ¼ teaspoon twice a day and graduate up to one teaspoon twice a day. If you can manage three times a day, even better!

- Use **spirulina powder** to replace all protein powders in smoothies.

- Include daily essential fatty acids like **Udo's Choice Blend** or **krill oil.**

- Make **PURE Better Butter** using half ghee and half organic coconut oil! This is great for sautés! Butter is a great fat. Learn to make ghee, and use as much of it as you like, whenever you want on "5 days" (unlimited). Be sure to always use organic.

- Include one serving of MUFA (monounsaturated fatty acid) foods with every meal. Choose from these MUFA foods:

    MUFA oils: flaxseed, olive, peanut, safflower, sesame, sunflower, or walnut. One serving equals one tablespoon.

    MUFA Nuts and Seeds: almonds, Brazil nuts, cashews, peanuts, sunflower seeds, hazelnuts, macadamia nuts, natural peanut butter, pecans, pine nuts, pistachios, pumpkin seeds, tahini (sesame seed paste), and walnuts. Macadamia is the best choice in this category. One serving of any of these is two tablespoons.

    Avocados: one serving equals ¼ cup.

    Olives: one serving equals ten olives or two tablespoons of tapenade (a spread made of chopped olives).

    Dark chocolate: one serving equals ¼ cup.

- Eat or juice **an apple a day**! Hey, you know what they say about apples... an apple a day keeps the doctor away!

- **Sugar-sweet Deception** — Use stevia or small amounts of honey, maple syrup, dates or date syrup as sweeteners. Nothing else! If you have blood sugar issues, want to reduce weight, or are trying to prevent or heal cancer, use stevia only.

Studies show the consumption of sugar leaves a broad range of consequences in its trail of continual usage. The toxic effects of sugar have been found to stimulate and aggravate these conditions:

Arthritis, appendicitis, asthma, atherosclerosis, candidiasis (yeast overgrowth), cancer (several types), constipation, coronary heart disease, Crohn's disease and ulcerative colitis, decreased growth hormone, depression and anxiety, diabetes, disturbed mineral balance, emphysema, eyesight issues, fatty liver, fluid retention, gallstones and kidney stones, kidney disease, headaches and migraines, hyperactivity, hormonal imbalances, multiple sclerosis, osteoporosis, speeds aging process, suppressed immunity, tooth decay and periodontal disease, weight gain and obesity.

Letting go of sugar is a huge step. I know the thought of not having that stimulation is scary for people who depend on it to make it through their day. However, you really will be pleasantly surprised to find that once you incorporate more and more raw foods and decrease cooked foods, especially grains, you will begin to experience real energy. The restored vitality, alertness, and spunk that comes from eating this way more than makes up for what you are restricting and ultimately relinquishing.

Quick Summary:

- Wean yourself off alcohol, sugar, all wheat, and all packaged and processed foods. For the 21 days see if you can restrict coffee and dairy.

- Get plenty of rest, regular exercise and moderate sunshine!

- Use your intuition on your "5 days" to eat as much or as little PURE food whenever you feel led to do so.

- The use of barley grass and spirulina is essential for maximum results. (See our websites listed in the Introduction and Chapter 6, *Get Eqipped* for ordering Organic Barley Grass and Spirulina.)

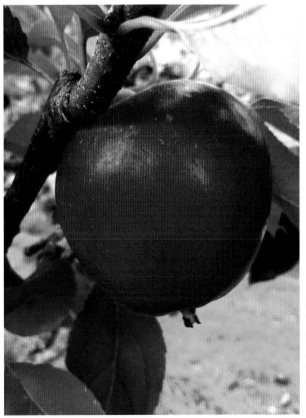

You know what they say about an apple a day...!

What Is Spirulina?

Spirulina is the botanical name of a blue-green algae that is barely half a millimeter long. In Latin the word Spirulina means little spiral, referring to the algae's spiral structure. Often referred to as the world's most nutritious natural superfood, spirulina contains the most remarkable concentration of nutrients known in any food, plant, grain or herb. It is the highest protein food—over 60% all-digestible vegetable protein. It has the highest concentration of beta-carotene, vitamin B12, iron and trace minerals and the rare essential fatty acid GLA.

Spirulina is a highly nutritious natural superfood for energy, maintaining health, weight loss and detox programs. This superfood is packed with essential fatty acids, protein, iron, calcium, vitamin B12 and vitamin E, chlorophyll, antioxidants, minerals and enzymes. The organic spirulina we offer is of the highest quality and potency, cultivated in a highly controlled environment to ensure purity.

Bring a little sunshine into your life:

Scientists have discovered that energy from the sun is extremely important for our health and is found mainly in fresh vegetables and sun-ripened fruit. Fresh Spirulina is a powerhouse that stores and converts enormous quantities of solar power into precious vitamins, minerals and energy.

Widely used as a food supplement for maintaining health, energy, weight loss and cleansing programs, spirulina is especially suitable for:

◆ **Athletes**: to improve performance, stamina and endurance and boost their high-energy lifestyle. For the bodybuilder, spirulina's most significant attribute is its high 65% easy-to-digest protein content.

◆ **Seniors**: for better digestion, increasing good health in the colon and relieving symptoms of constipation. As a highly nutritious and easily digested food, spirulina also has a beneficial effect on malabsorption, a common problem for seniors.

◆ **Pregnant and nursing mothers:** providing extra protein and iron, without the additional fats and carbohydrates.

◆ **Those following a weight loss plan:** to support a healthy balanced diet, Spirulina is a highly concentrated natural food that helps to restore natural body weight by satisfying the body's real hunger for nutrition.

Organic Barley Grass

Barley grass juice powder provides a super-store of vitamins, minerals and enzymes for everyday vitality and well-being. This remarkable juice also contains all nine essential amino acids, which help our body's cells to function optimally.

The barley grass juice powder we offer is certified organic and juiced immediately after harvesting. It is low-temperature carbon dioxide dried to ensure that it contains the highest possible levels of enzymes, chlorophyll and other nutrients. Simply add to water to enjoy an instant fresh juice or add to your favorite smoothie!

PURE treats – After about three weeks, sugar stops calling you and real, pure food takes on new flavors and meaning. You will find that your body's cravings will disappear and you will know satisfaction from the nourishment your body is receiving. Your palate will come back to life and eating a piece of fruit will become a simple, yet fulfilling dessert. You can still allow yourself the opportunity to enjoy sweets, once in a while. Sweets become a conscious treat that you intuitively know won't upset your balance. Eaten with awareness and made with PURE ingredients, PURE treats can be just the thing to help create balance and moderation, making the PURE 5:2 lifestyle very sustainable. We included a great Raw Chocolate recipe — see page 159!

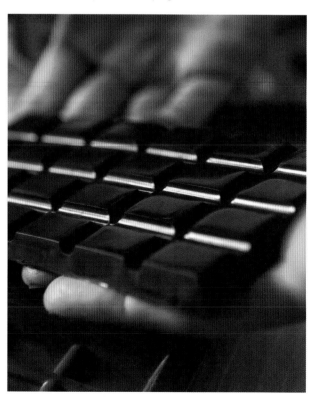

Raw chocolate by Rosie the Chocolate Chica!

Drink any combination of liquids listed (in the Beverage section) throughout the day. Break the fast any time between 16–24 hours from your last meal, unless you feel intuitively to break it sooner. Listen to your body and be sure to nourish yourself well with PURE liquids and foods. Ideally break the fast with PURE revival foods (see recipes). Pay attention to glycemic load and stay away from sugars, sugary drinks and carbs that will quickly turn to sugar.

NOTE: It is essential on "2 days" to keep your blood sugar from spiking. If you have blood sugar issues or notice you spike too much from drinking fresh juice or find you can't go for very long without food, try adding a heaping tablespoon of coconut oil into your juice and mix well in a blender.

Break the fast with a dinner that includes balanced proteins and healthy fats. Add spirulina into your drinks during the day for extra protein, vitamins and minerals. Nibble on greens and raw vegetables towards the later afternoon and even have a plate of sautéed or steamed greens. In the later afternoon you can also snack on Kale Chips (see the recipe on page 141).

◆ Begin each day adding the juice of one lemon to 16–32 ounces of warm water and drink first thing in the morning. This will help to move bowels, cleanse kidneys and urinary tract, alkalize the body, kick-start the liver, remove mucus, and hydrate the body. (Optional: add 1 teaspoon Manuka honey or honey with cayenne pepper.)

◆ Drink barley powder in water, apple juice diluted with water, coconut water, or carrot juice (start with ¼ teaspoon and work up to one teaspoon 2–3 times a day)

◆ Make a high nutrient density smoothie with spirulina and fresh spinach or kale (see PURE Break-Fast Smoothie on page 95)

◆ Make a potassium flush broth, Bieler's Broth, or bone broth (your choice). Have as much as you like throughout the day. (See broth recipes, pages 109 and 110)

◆ Make a pitcher of lemon water or vitamin/mineral water

◆ Drink one or more cups of warm high antioxidant, detox, or cleansing tea (see tea suggestions, page 103)

◆ Make and drink fresh juice (see juice recipes, pages 105-107)

*PURE "2 Days" – Easy Option: PURE "2 days" can be made very easy by using the following two products:

1. **PHP's Power Shake**™ (*NOTE:* available in Europe as **Hippokrates Power Powder**) was created so that you can easily consume several PURE, organic, superfoods all at once, ready to go, thus saving you time and money. For detoxification, we recommend using the Power Shake as part of your "2 days." Comes in original and new apple berry flavors. Mix the Power Shake powder with water or juice and drink for breakfast lunch and dinner on your "2 days."

The Power Shake: (either flavor)
   ◆ is a great natural detoxifier
   ◆ may help burn fat and build muscle
   ◆ may increase energy, endurance, and strength
   ◆ supports healthy blood glucose levels
   ◆ can help curb cravings and appetite
   ◆ contains ingredients rich in vitamins and nutrients to support total nutrition

2. **PHP Apothe-Cherry**™ is made from Montmorency Tart Cherries, which are nature's most nutritionally dense food. They contain a wide variety of antioxidants and phyto-chemicals, and each serving contains 7,000 ORAC (Oxygen Radical Absorbance Capacity) units. We recommend adding ½ to one ounce (1–2 tablespoons) of concentrate to 8–10 ounces of water or juice. Works best when taken thirty minutes to an hour before going to bed or after a workout.
   ◆ Contains melatonin, which may help balance circadian rhythms for proper sleep
   ◆ May support healthy joint function
   ◆ Promotes healthy uric acid metabolism
   ◆ Is a rich source of antioxidants
   ◆ Can help prevent or even reverse premature aging

To order these products, visit:
USA: **phporder.com/rawsome**
Europe: **platinumuk.biz/rawsome**

PURE 5:2 Essentials for Transformation Success

For these 21 days of transformation **restrict** (hold back from eating) these foods:

✗ **Wheat in any form**
✗ **All sugar in all forms unless otherwise stated**
✗ **All processed and packaged foods**
✗ **Grains, except for oats groats and quinoa (and only use these very sparingly)**

Eat as much raw as possible. The enzymes in raw foods are a key for digestive health as well as for anti-aging benefits including being a catalyst for antioxidant and anti-inflammatory effects.

Eliminate dairy, except small amounts of goat yogurt and raw goat cheese.

Use of good fats is unrestricted. Make sure all oils, nuts, seeds, and especially butter are organic, as chemicals bond to fats. Eat only organic grass-fed meat and free-range eggs. Buy only wild fish. Add MUFA fats such as olives and avocados to each meal (see page 57 for MUFA fats description).

Modified Intermittent Fasting for Blood Sugar Regulation

For various reasons, you may need to modify intermittent fasting. The most obvious reason is for blood sugar regulation. That being the case, we suggest 21 days of no grains, sugars, alcohol or dairy except butter and goat yogurt.

Restrict eating to smaller portions 4 times a day. Drink lemon water upon arising, before every meal, and throughout the day. Have quality protein and fat at every meal. Eat PURE vegetables and low-glycemic fruits if any fruits at all. Use organic nuts and seeds, olive oil and coconut oil. Especially emphasize freshly ground linseeds/flax seeds, chia seeds and walnuts* for their beneficial omega oils, helpful in combating metabolic disease.

Drink fresh vegetable juices, and mix in coconut oil whenever you include carrots and beets in your juice, to slow down how their sugar is metabolized. Include spirulina and barley grass. Make and drink nourishing broths as often as possible. Add homemade whey into your drinks and soups (when not too hot). If you choose to include raw eggs in smoothies for quality protein, boil water and dip the egg in for a few seconds. Then rinse under cold water before opening. Use only stevia and cinnamon for sweetening.

Another Highly Effective Approach to Intermittent Fasting

Another approach for many people that brings fantastic results is to only eat during a window of approximately 6–8 hours. Ideally, it is best to stop eating past 7pm at night and to continue to restrict eating until after 11am in the morning. This form of intermittent fasting, where one skips breakfast, has been scientifically proven to yield incredibly beneficial results, such as improving insulin sensitivity and shifting into burning more fat instead of sugar for fuel.

As your body shifts into the new ability to burn fat, the result is painless weight loss without the dreaded hunger pangs and imbalanced blood sugar swings. To "break-the-fast" you begin with warm lemon water and move on to fresh raw vegetable juice (great to include barley grass with that). With the window of eating between 11am and 7pm, you can then eat unrestricted, PURE food. Some people make this their daily regime. By fasting daily for 16–18 hours, this is enough to get your body to shift into fat-burning mode. This style of fasting yields great results, and therefore makes it a compelling alternative.

Intermittent fasting does not have to mean two days of restricted eating and five days unrestricted. Rather it refers to periods of time where food is restricted for extended periods of time. This can be a gradual process so you can ease your way into it without a jolt. You can start by not eating anything

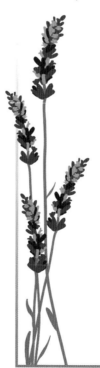

Once a week, sit in a really warm bath that contains a handful of Epsom or sea salts, 10 drops of lavender essential oil, and a half cup of baking soda for at least 20 minutes.

This combo aids in drawing out toxins, lowering stress-related hormones and balancing your pH levels.

three hours prior to going to sleep. Wait as long as you can to "break" the fast. Gradually, one day at a time, increase the amount of time you wait until "breaking the fast" until you are able to restrict eating for 16–18 hours at a stretch. Ideally, try to eat your first meal at lunchtime.

This approach also works well as a continuation once you end your PURE 5:2 Transformation in 21 Days. Personally, I found this approach to be a natural next step and I LOVE the results. It takes only a few weeks to adjust to this approach. Once you shift into fat burning mode, science has proven the following list of potential benefits:

We want to encourage you to be creative, work at your own pace and experiment by listening to your own body and unique needs. Use your intuition to create the 5:2 plan that works best for you.

◆ Normalizing insulin sensitivity, imperative for optimal health, as insulin resistance is a primary contributing factor to nearly all chronic disease, from diabetes to heart disease, as well as cancer

◆ Normalizing ghrelin levels ("the hunger hormone")

◆ Promoting human growth hormone (HGH) production, which is vital in health, fitness and slowing the aging process

◆ Lowering triglyceride levels

◆ Reducing inflammation and lessening free-radical damage

*Lifestyle Counseling and Supplementation with Flaxseed or Walnuts Influence the Management of Metabolic Syndrome 1–4; American Society for Nutrition, 2010.

PURE 5:2 Transformation and Beyond

Old habits are transformed not by self-coercion, but by attraction to fresh awareness along with intentional choices, producing an awakened sense of aliveness.

We feel confident that 21 days is enough time for you to put into practice PURE 5:2 so that you will absolutely feel the transformation. Once you feel the difference, the choice to continue becomes clear. The awakened sense of aliveness and delight from truly learning and mastering how to nourish yourself well creates a momentum to carry on. The results and rewards are endless! You might find it quite easy to naturally shift over to the alternative approach mentioned in the previous section. This suggested approach works wonderfully as an easy-to-apply daily regime. We would love to hear your success stories. Please do write to us and let us know how this has impacted you. **Eat well and be well!**

Robyn and Geoff Randolph

purehighlandliving@gmail.com

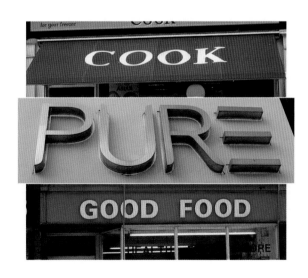

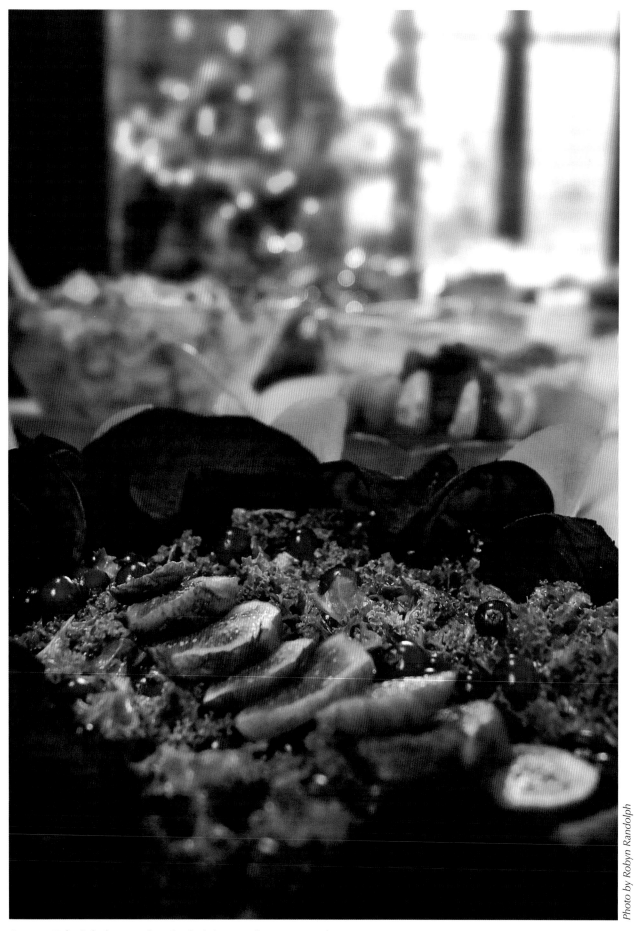

Festive Kale Salad — perfect for holiday meals! Recipe on page 126.

PART 2
CHAPTER 5

Nutrient-dense Recipes for PURE Transformation in 21 Days

In this section, we provide a range of recipe ideas to assist in your 21 day PURE Transformation. For more recipe ideas see my book *RawSome Recipes* (found on Amazon USA), or for free recipes go to our websites:

www.purehighlandliving.com
www.kaleconsciousness.com

or type in our channel: **Pure Highland Living** on YouTube.com to watch our videos.

Whether you are a vegan, vegetarian, or carnivore, the recipes in this book emphasize mostly Raw with Some cooked foods (RawSome), so as to get maximum enzymes into your daily diet. Most everyone we meet needs help and inspiration to incorporate more raw, PURE food into their diet.

"Two days" are an opportunity to eat mostly raw and restrain from animal products and cooked foods. Eating mostly raw helps the body to detox, cleanse and benefit from the enzymes that get destroyed in cooking.

Use your intuition whether or not to add quality grass-fed, organic animal products into your "five days" as appropriate and for your individual needs.

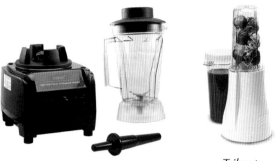

Enpee Blender

Tribest
Personal Blender

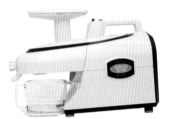

Tribest Elite Juicer

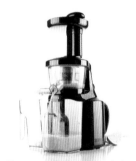

Enpee Masticating Juicer

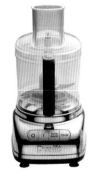

Dualit Food Processor

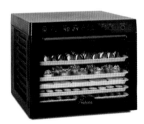

Tribest Sedona
Dehydrator

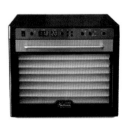

NEW Tribest Sedona
Combo Digital Dehydrator

About Our Tools

Recipes requiring special equipment will have icons of our favorite blender(s), food processor, juicers, or dehydrator(s) — see key at the bottom of this column. If you already have this equipment, it is great to use what you already have as long as it gets the job done. We are here to assist if you need help getting equipped or upgrading.

We enjoy using the commercial-grade blender by Enpee, as well as the convenient Personal Blender by Tribest (for smaller recipes such as salad dressings, or grinding nuts or linseeds). It is lovely to have the power of the commercial blender for big bulky items that require a strong motor and for mixing large quantities of ingredients. The Personal Blender makes life easy when it comes to convenience, travel, and clean-up.

Our favorite juicer is The Elite, made by Tribest, because it produces the absolute highest-quality juice. However, we really like also providing the Enpee Masticating Juicer for those who want a more affordable juicer with a sturdy motor that produces good quality juice. We like how easy this juicer is to set up and to clean.

Since moving to Scotland, we have discovered the Dualit Food Processor, which is by far the best we have ever used.

The Sedona Dehydrator set the standard being the first dehydrator on the market using BPA-free plastic, a very big step in the right direction for reducing obesogens from our food. The new model (shown on right) includes a digital two-stage sequential temperature-timer, which enables you to kickstart the dehydration process at a higher temperature and then automatically lower the temperature to finish off the process. Great for fruits and veggies with a high water content, and reduces the overall dehydrating time.

We sell this equipment both in the USA and the UK, except the Dualit Food Processor, Enpee blender and Enpee juicer, which are only available in the UK. For USA, if you don't see a price for the equipment you want please contact us.

To see our full range and how to order go to Chapter 6, *Get Equipped.*

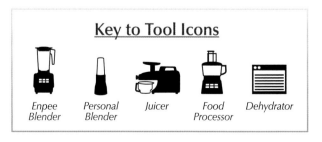

Key to Tool Icons

Enpee
Blender

Personal
Blender

Juicer

Food
Processor

Dehydrator

Conversions

Below you will find general guides for the approximate conversions of Imperial measurements to metric. All of the recipes in this book are very forgiving so do not worry if you don't measure in exact amounts. You can always add or subtract according to your own intuitive taste buds!

Volume		Dry Weight
1 teaspoon = 5ml	1oz = 30ml	1oz = 30 g
2 teaspoons = 10ml	2oz = 60ml	2oz = 60g
1 tablespoon = 15ml	3oz = 85ml	3oz = 90g
2 tablespoons = 30ml	4oz = 120ml	4oz = 120g
	5oz = 140m	5oz = 150g

Welcome to Real People, Pure Food…

from the heart of the Highlands! This is a collection of photos from some of our farm-to-table cooking adventures with our Scottish community of friends, intuitive chefs and farmers.

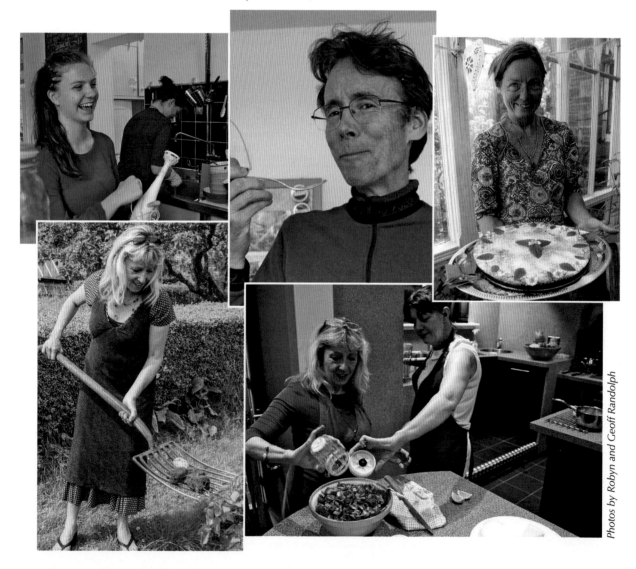

Photos by Robyn and Geoff Randolph

Together we share a passion for growing and preparing PURE Food!

You are invited to join us in our Pure Food Revival! If you are interested in attending a PURE Healthy Holiday Retreat, workshop or PURE personalized food coaching contact us:

purehighlandliving@gmail.com

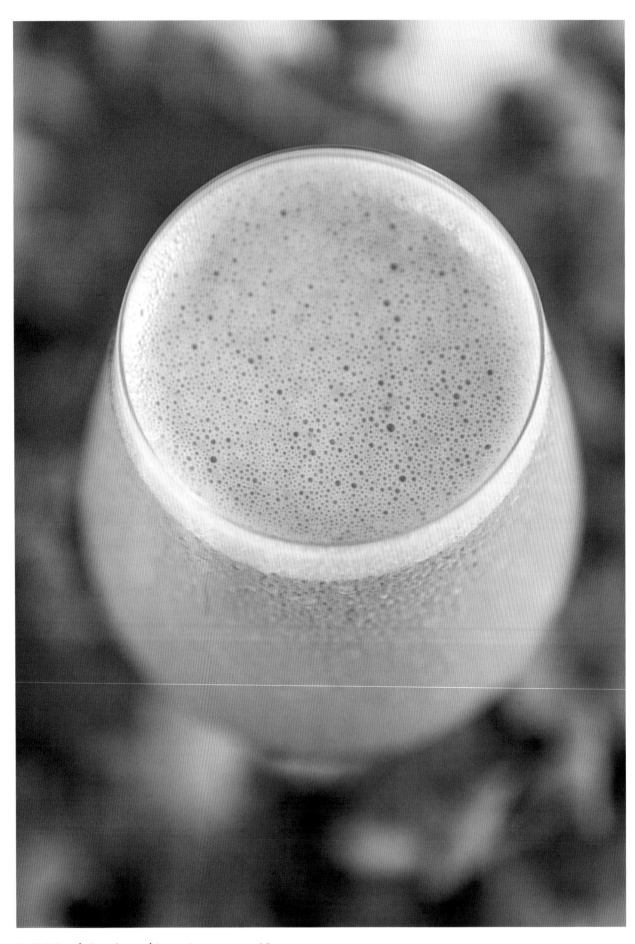

PURE Break-Fast Smoothie, recipe on page 95.

92

Warm Lemon Water

Start each day with warm lemon water. Lemons are a great way to cleanse and alkalinize. Additionally lemon water is a great natural appetite suppressant.

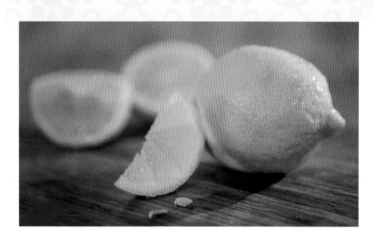

  8 ounces water
  Juice of one lemon
  Manuka honey (optional)
  Cayenne pepper (optional)

1. Boil water and put 4 ounces hot water in mug.

2. Add 4 ounces cold water.

3. Now add lemon juice (having the water warm, not hot, will keep the enzymes in the lemon intact).

Barley Grass Juice

The great thing about barley grass juice is no blender or juicer is required because it comes in a convenient enzyme-packed, raw powder that can be mixed and stirred into liquids. Barley grass is a great thing to pack along when you are away from home. It is easy to transport and use when you are on the run. Mix in a shaker bottle or jar with a tight lid when you are on the go or use a blender to avoid clumping. Start with ¼ tsp. and then a few days later shift to ½ tsp. Do that a few days and then move up to ¾ tsp. and then finally move to 1 tsp three times a day. Mix well.

Optimally it is great to incorporate 1 tsp. barley grass two or three times per day, everyday. Barley grass is a detoxifier, blood purifier and immune system builder. Your cells will love you for it! If you like the taste of freshly mowed grass then water will do, but otherwise I suggest coconut water, apple juice or fresh carrot juice. See Chapter 6, *Get Equipped,* for how to order barley grass.

NOTE: Barley grass juice does NOT contain any gluten. People often assume it does because the grain of barley DOES contain gluten. The fresh young grass is much like wheat grass and both grasses without the seed are 100% gluten free.

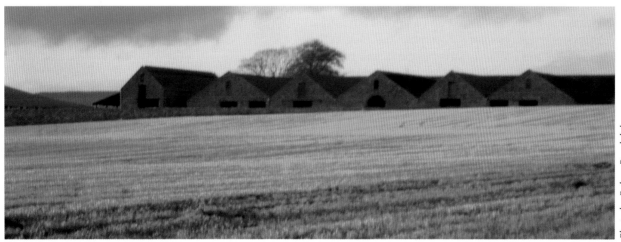

Photo by Robyn Randolph

Scottish barley field – the grains in this photo are not to be confused with gluten-free barley grass.

Barley Blast

> ¼ – 1 tsp. barley grass powder
> 8 ounces water, apple juice, coconut water or fresh carrot juice

Mix all together in personal blender or Enpee Blender (See Chapter 6, *Get Equipped,* to order barley grass powder or tools).

Crème de Barley Blast

Recently, on a "2 day," I had come in from a brisk walk on the beach and was feeling quite peckish. I had several hours to go until breaking the fast and knew if I drank straight carrot juice I would spike my blood sugar too much. After asking myself what I needed in that moment, I intuitively was inspired to add ½ of a small avocado with 1 teaspoon of barley grass into fresh carrot juice. It was one of those ah-ha moments that hit the target, spot-on and yielded the exact results my body was requesting! Delicious, nutritious and the fat in the avocado helped slow down the sugar in the carrot juice so my pancreas was not inundated. This has become a new personal favorite afternoon drink delight for a "2 day." Try it and let me know what you think. Especially for all you low blood sugar types that love a little carrot juice from time to time!

> ¼ – 1 tsp. barley grass powder (see *Get Equipped*)
> 8 ounces fresh carrot juice
> ½ small avocado or you could substitute this with ½ – 1 T. coconut oil

Homemade Almond Milk Made in the Soyabella

Fresh almond milk is our favorite nutritious non-dairy alternative. Almond milk provides magnesium, potassium and vitamin E. The ratio of calcium to protein is almost identical to that of human breast milk. It is lower in calories than regular milk and a great choice for people with milk allergies.

When you make homemade almond milk the leftover pulp can be used for baking, raw pie crusts, pates, and dehydrated crackers.

We used to make our almond milk using a "nut bag." It was messy and time consuming, so we tended not to do it that often. We depended on store-bought almond milk until we realized that the ingredients in manufactured almond milk were not so great on a daily basis. Then we discovered the fabulous Soyabella machine. Now making almond milk is a snap and literally takes seconds. All you do is fill the Soyabella container up with water to the watermark line. Pop one cup of soaked almonds into the inner container. Assemble and plug in the machine and hit the milling button. It will process the almonds for about 15 seconds and shut off. Hit the button for two more cycles and that is it! Done. In less than a minute you have delicious fresh almond milk.

Pour it into a glass pitcher and store it in the fridge. Save and use the pulp. Clean up is a snap. It is that easy! (Go to **purehighlandlivng.com** if you would like to order a Soyabella.)

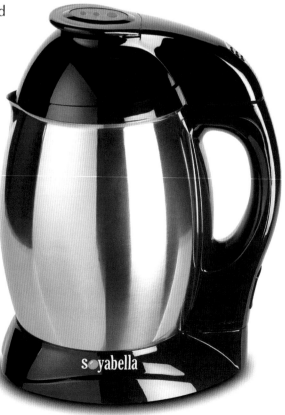

Photo courtesy of Tribest Corporation

Sweet Almond Milk

> 2–4 pitted dates
> 1 tsp. vanilla
> 1 tsp. cinnamon
> Pinch of Himalayan salt

1. Make fresh almond milk as suggested in the Soybella.
2. Pour milk into blender with all of the above ingredients and blend on high.
3. Pour into a glass pitcher and store in the fridge.

Coconut Vanilla Mystic

> 2 cups fresh almond milk
> 1 heaping T. organic coconut oil
> 1 tsp. vanilla powder or 1 vanilla pod,
>   snipped into small bits
> 2 tsp. agave nectar, date syrup
>   or maple syrup
> Pinch of Himalayan salt
> 1 T. spirulina powder (optional)
>   (see Chapter 6, *Get Equipped,* for
>   how to order)

Liquify all ingredients in blender on high speed for at least two minutes.

PURE Break-Fast Smoothie

Great for "5 Days"

> 1 T. flax seed – grind alone in blender
>   or coffee grinder
> 1 banana fresh or frozen (optional)
> 1 T. spirulina (see *Get Equipped*)
> 1 big handful raw spinach
> 1 apple, cut in chunks for blender
> 1 cup almond milk, goat milk,
>   coconut water, coconut milk or
>   pure water
> 1–2 T. organic walnuts and/or 1 T.
>   coconut oil or ½ avocado
> 1–2 T. fresh homemade whey
>   (optional)
> 2 T. goat yogurt (optional)
> 1 raw egg (optional)
> 1 T. raisins or 2 pitted dates (optional)

Blend starting slow and then gradually move to high speed. Serves 1.

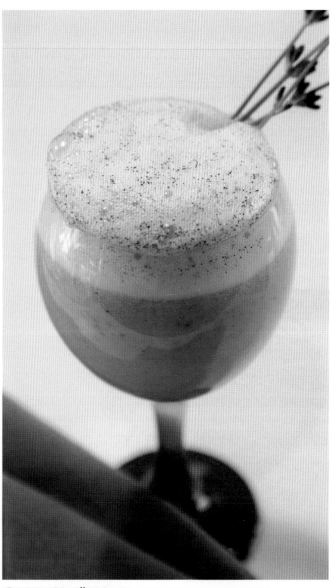

Coconut Vanilla Mystic

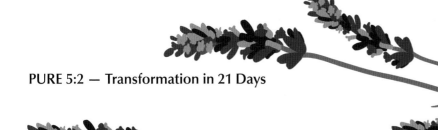

Banana Carob Mint Spirulina Smoothie

 2 cups or 250ml almond milk, goat milk, coconut milk or combo of these
 4 organic walnuts
 1 T. chia seeds
 1 banana fresh or frozen (optional)
 1 T. carob mint spirulina (see Chapter 6, *Get Equipped,* for how to order)
 4 leaves fresh mint
 2 big leaves of kale
 2 big leaves of beet greens
 1 apple, cut in chunks for blender
 ¼ tsp. vanilla

Blend starting slow and then gradually move to high speed.
Serves 1–2.

Banana Coconut Cream Smoothie (Great for "5 Days")

 8 oz. coconut milk, almond milk, goat's milk, water or combo of any of these
 ½–1 frozen banana
 1 T. of coconut oil (helps slow down the impact of the banana sugar)
 1 heaping T. spirulina (carob mint is our favorite made by PHP for USA only, see *Get Equipped*)
 4–6 walnuts
 2 handfuls of clean spinach
 1 raw egg (optional)
 ½ avocado (great fat that works well with the impact of the banana)
 1 tsp. cinnamon (helps regulate blood sugar)

Blend starting slow and then gradually move to high speed. Serves 2.

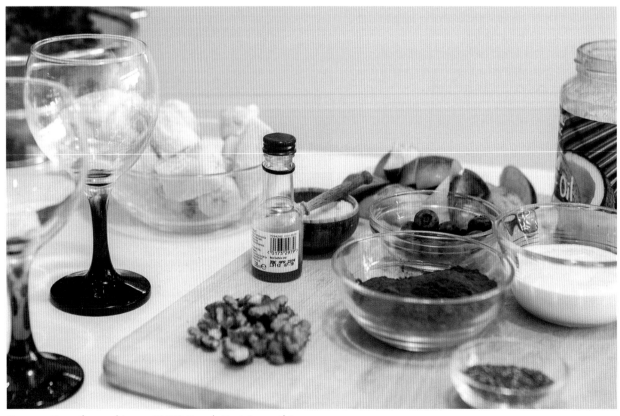

Preparations for making a PURE Break-Fast Smoothie.

Blueberry Banana-Fanna Smoothie (Great for "5 Days")

8 oz. coconut milk, almond milk, goat's milk, water or combo of any of these
½–1 frozen banana
1 T. of coconut oil (helps slow down the impact of the banana sugar)
1 heaping T. spirulina (carob mint is our favorite — see *Get Equipped*)
½–¾ cup fresh or frozen blueberries (or any combination of berries)

Blend starting slow and then gradually move to high speed. Serves 1.

PURE Smoothie for "2 Days"

1 T. spirulina (see *Get Equipped* for how to order)
2 handfuls raw spinach
1 apple, cut in chunks for blender
¾–1 cup pure water
½–1 tsp. cinnamon
Tiny amount of stevia (to taste)
Vanilla or organic raw cocoa powder (to taste)

Blend starting slow and then gradually move to high speed. Serves 1.

Creamy Cashew Milk

The wonderful thing about cashew milk, as opposed to almond milk, is that there is no nut bag or straining required. This is especially true if you have a heavy duty blender like the Enpee. This is such a yummy milk to use in teas, smoothies or on porridge.

1½ cups cashews
4 cups water
4 dates
1 T. cooks vanilla or 1 vanilla powder
½ tsp. cinnamon

Liquefy all ingredients in blender on high speed for at least two minutes. Serves 4.

OPTION: For a richer milk, add 3 tsp. coconut oil.

Coconut Mango Lassi

Orange, creamy and refreshing.

2 cups organic orange juice
1 frozen banana
8–10 pieces frozen mango chunks
2 heaping T. coconut oil

1. Cut mango into cubes and freeze overnight.

2. Blend on high until you have a thick, creamy lassi. Great afternoon snack on a warm day! Serves 2.

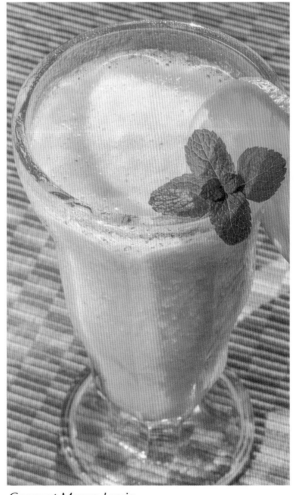

Coconut Mango Lassie

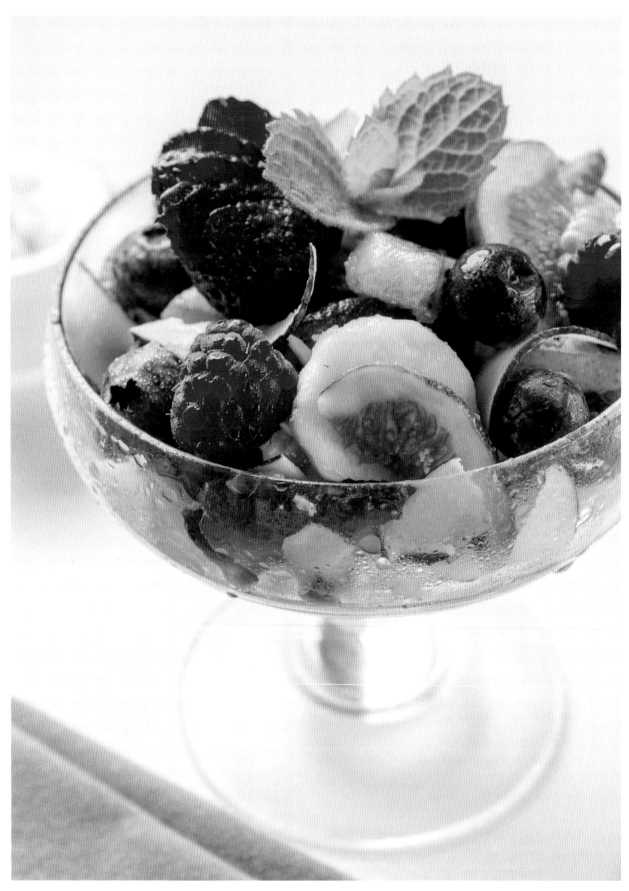

Morning Medley of Fresh Fruit

Use any amount of fresh shaved coconut meat with raspberries, figs, blueberries, strawberries, pears and bananas. Garnish with fresh mint.

Banana Cardamom Milkshake (or Ice Cream)

If you like the popular Indian spice, cardamom, you will LOVE this!

Seeds of 2 crushed cardamom pods
½ cup coconut milk, almond milk or cashew milk
(more or less, depending on if you want a milkshake or ice cream)
3 or 4 frozen bananas
½ tsp. vanilla powder or snip in one vanilla pod

Liquefy all ingredients in blender on high speed. Serves 2.

Coconut Chia Pineapple Passion Porridge/Pudding

Intuitive cooking is fun, freeing and forgiving. Just tune in and you will "know" what amounts of what to use depending on your personal tastes and unique nutritional requirements at the time. This recipes is refreshing, delicious, raw and really easy! (See photo of recipe on page 14.)

Soak ½–1 cup of chia seeds with more than enough liquid to cover (approx. 2–2½ cups liquid to every ½ cup of chia). Use pineapple juice and/or coconut water combined. I like a strong pineapple accent so I used a ratio of about 3/4 pineapple and 1/4 coconut juice (sometimes just one or the other).

Add a handful of shredded coconut and 1–2 T. date syrup with a pinch of Himalayan salt. Stir vigorously, making sure everything is blended and bathed in the liquid. You can also use stevia or fruit juice-sweetened apricot jam.

Set on counter and come back and stir again from time to time. You can place in fridge and let set, however this is best served room temp.

Put into small dessert bowls or cups and top with fresh passion fruit and light sprinkles of shredded coconut.

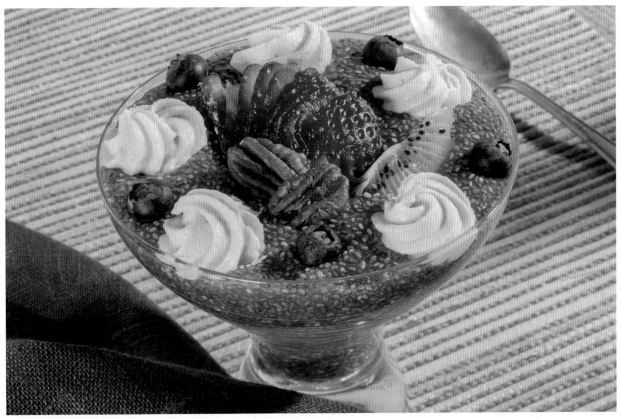

OPTION: Coconut cream or cashew milk work well as a decorative topping with passion fruit. Or come up with your own "intuitive topping." Here is one I made with what I had on hand.

Good Morning Granola!

This is a great recipe for people who are gluten free and avoiding grains. We love to eat this mixture, raw from the mixing bowl, before it even gets dehydrated (the flavors are that good)! Serve with homemade almond or cashew milk.

2 cups almonds, soaked 12 hours in a separate bowl
½ cup each: pumpkin seeds, sunflower seeds, pecans and walnuts all soaked
4 hours (soak seeds in one bowl and nuts in another)
2 cups apples
1 T. cinnamon
1 T. vanilla
1 tsp. Himalayan salt
sliced strawberries
½ cup shredded dried coconut

1. Rinse and drain nuts and seeds.

2. With the "S" blade of a processor, begin chunking down the almonds into small bits. Empty contents into a big mixing bowl.

3. Repeat processing with the pumpkin and sunflower seeds until all are small chunky bits, not over-processing. Add to almonds and repeat process using the shredding device.

4. Next core and cut apples into quarters. Put through processor using the shredding device.

5. Mix all ingredients together except for the coconut and cut strawberries.

6. Using a drying sheet, spread the granola onto tray, making sure not to mound it.

7. Sprinkle the sliced strawberries evenly on the tray. Dehydrate up to 24 hours at 117°F or 47°C until granola is crisp and crunchy.

8. Mix the dried granola in with the coconut and store in tall glass jars for maximum shelf life. If your granola seems stale or damp as time goes on, you can try re-dehydrating it, which generally perks it right up again!

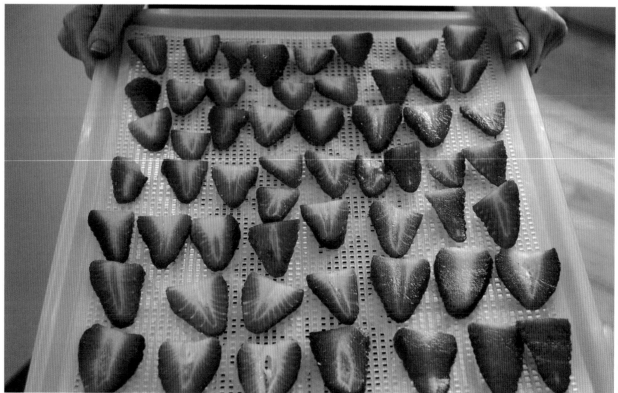

Photo by Robyn Randolph

Sometimes I like to dehydrate a tray of strawberries and have them ready to mix in at the end, when the granola is done.

Vitamin/Mineral Waters

Cucumber Water

1 quart of water
1 English cucumber, sliced thin
Cucumber Water
1 lime, sliced thin
Dill, basil, mint sprigs, or borage flowers

Pineapple Water

1 quart water
⅓ pineapple, sliced in thin triangular wedges
Spearmint, lemon balm, mint, borage or
    lavender flowers

Melon Water

1 quart water
2 cups thin triangular wedges of
    watermelon, honeydew or cantaloupe
1 lime, sliced very thin
Lavender sprigs or mint (optional)

Berry Water

1 quart water
2 cups of any or all of these: raspberries,
    strawberries, blueberries or blackberries
1 lemon, sliced thin
Borage flowers or leaves, sweet mint

Citrus Cooler

1 quart water
1 each: lemon, lime and orange
3 slices of ginger (optional)
Edible flowers to float on the surface

Parsley Refresher

1 quart water
1 sliced lemon
Handful of Italian flat-leaf parsley leaves

A great palate cleanser at meals!

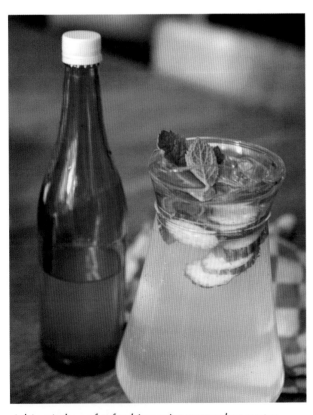

A big pitcher of refreshing mint cucumber water.

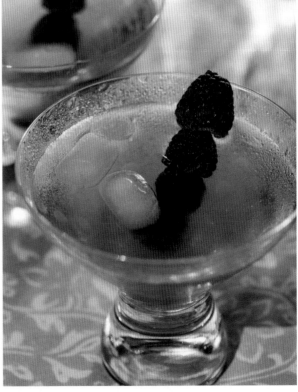

Dress up a glass of berry water with fresh berries or edible flowers

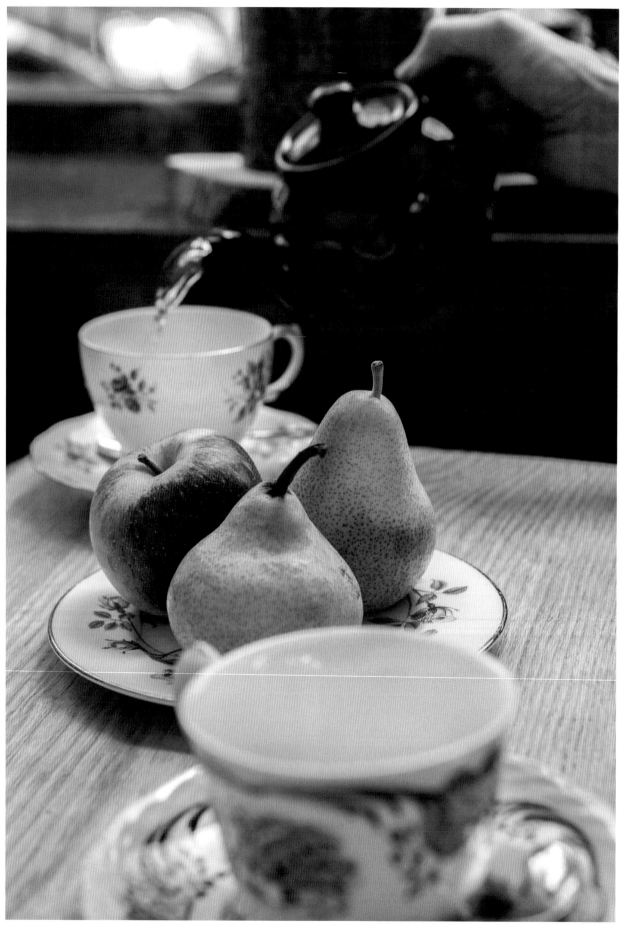

Enjoying a spot of organic afternoon tea at Velocity Cafe in Inverness, Scotland.

Tea

Cleanse, Nourish, Balance Tea Blend

Peppermint
Fennel
Nettles
Oat-straw
Alfalfa
Licorice (optional)
Chamomile

1. Combine equal amounts of the dried herbs in a canning jar (with a tight fitting lid) and store until needed.
2. Fill cloth tea bag or tea strainer and steep to desired strength.
3. To make a pot of tea, fill saucepan with enough water for the pot.
4. Boil water and turn off heat.
5. Add loose tea, 2–4 heaping tablespoons. Cover and let steep.
6. Strain and fill teapot.
7. Fill a glass jar or thermos and sip on this tea all day if you want!

Creamy Cardamom and Turmeric Tea

1 cup almond, hazelnut or coconut milk
½ tsp. turmeric
½ tsp. cardamom
½ inch wide slice of ginger, minced
1 tsp. manuka honey or date syrup
¼ tsp. cinnamon or nutmeg

1. Warm the milk in pan, not too hot.
2. Add all ingredients and stir well.
3. Strain when pouring into cup.

Immuni-Tea

Great for busting your immune system, and especially good for winter days. By Claire MacKay of Herbal Heritage Scotland: www.herbalheritage.co.uk

Echinacea
Elderflower
Nettle
Calendula
Borage

Combine in any amounts.

Our Favorite Commercially Available Teas

Tulsi or Holy Basil Tea

Widely known in India as a powerful antioxidant recognized and used for these benefits:

◆ Enhancing respiratory system
◆ Supporting healthy vision
◆ Antioxidant protection against free radicals
◆ Calming and soothing effect great for stress relief
◆ Immune system booster
◆ Helping you promote a healthy metabolism
◆ Supports digestive system health
◆ Helps to maintain normal blood sugar levels
◆ Providing skeletal and joint support
◆ Maintaining normal cholesterol levels

Rooibos

High-antioxidant tea without caffeine.

Green Tea

High-antioxidant tea, great for those trying to wean off coffee.

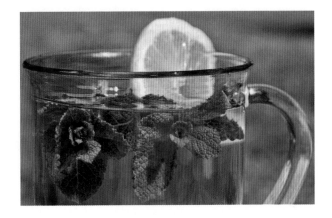

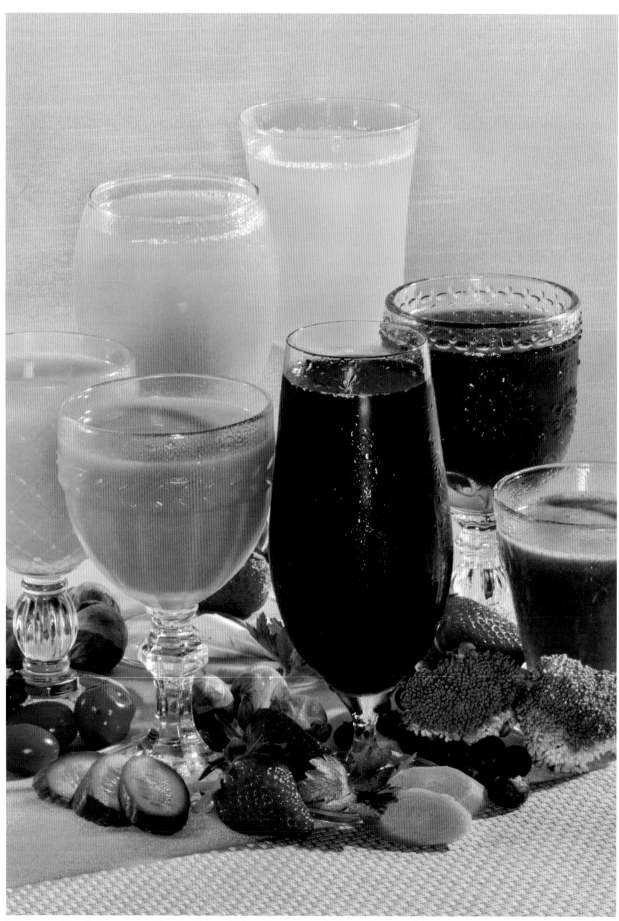

When making juices, a good rule of thumb is to keep your fruits and vegetables separate. Exceptions are apples, lemons, and limes.

Juices

Blood Purifying Fruits and Vegetables

The following exceptional foods are excellent choices for adding to smoothies or juicing as their detoxifying and blood purifying properties make them super detox foods:

Apples, spinach, strawberries, limes, dates, raisins, beetroot, bell peppers, mangos, kale, tomato, broccoli, cabbage, and prunes

How do these foods help to detox and purify the blood? The fiber in these foods, adds bulk to the feces and helps to stimulate the digestive process. This results in reduced transit time of the stool, exposing the colon to fewer carcinogens. Fiber aids in the removal of accumulated, waste matter, thus purifying the blood.

Additionally, insoluble fiber provides good bacteria, which is an important contributing factor for maintaining a healthy colon.

These foods contain phytochemicals with potent anti-oxidant properties useful as protection against free radical damage and prevention against diseases.

NOTE: A little-known fact is that raisins have been shown to have antibacterial properties that help prevent plaque on teeth. We like to use raisins to sweeten recipes, including smoothies, as a nice alternative to other forms of sweeteners.

Red Revival Juice

This is the PURE 5:2 signature juice for our workshops! Wait until you try this! You will taste and feel why.

Purple cabbage is a phytochemical food containing a powerful anti-oxidant called "anthocyanin."

This juice is an anti-oxidant with anti-inflammatory effect, wonderful for relieving inflammation like gout, arthritis and joint pains. Great preventative juice for the risks of breast, colon, liver, lung and ovarian cancers. Also restorative to the digestive tract as well as boosting the immune system.

> 4 apples, cut in slices
>   for the juicer
> 1 large red beet
> 1 whole lime, skin and all
> 1-inch knuckle of ginger
> ¼ small purple cabbage
> 1 tsp. barley grass powder stirred in once
>   everything is juiced (optional)

Juice everything together and drink up!
Serves 1–2.

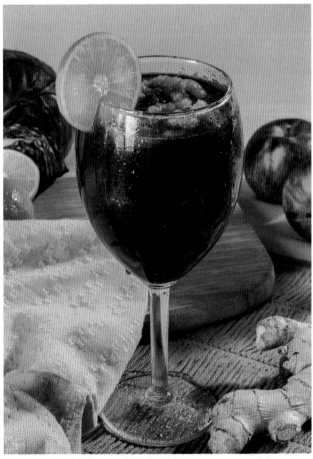

This is the PURE 5:2 signature juice for our workshops!

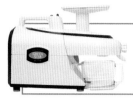

NOTE: The recipes on these two pages all require a juicer. (See Chapter 6, *Get Equipped,* for the ones we recommend).

Kale and Cabbage Calcium Boost

2–4 green apples, cut in slices for the juicer
Intuitive amounts of kale and spinach
Beet top greens
1 cup green cabbage

Makes approximately 2 servings of juice.

Simply Apple/Pear

2 organic apples
2 organic pears

1. Wash and slice up pears and apples.
2. Put through juicer.
3. Pour juice through a fine mesh strainer and enjoy!

Makes approximately 2 servings of juice.

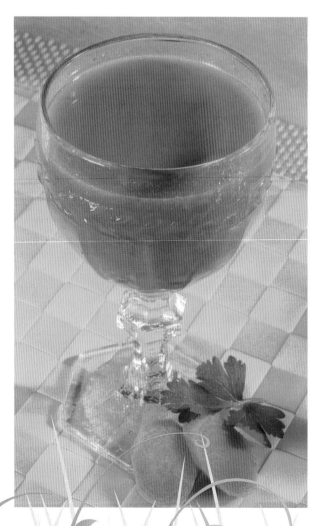

Intuitive Lean Green Juice

Intuitive amounts of:
Celery
Cucumber
Spinach
Kale
Green apples

Sunshine Juice

1 large pineapple, juiced
2–4 oranges
Carrot juice (optional)

Makes approximately 2 servings of juice.

Carrot Clarity

4 green apples
8 large carrots
1 large cucumber
Fresh ginger knuckle, 1–2 inches

Makes approximately 2 servings of juice.

Creamy Carrot Ginger Juice

(This recipe also requires a blender)

This is super delicious and the coconut oil gives you immediate fuel and energy. A wonderful juice for people with blood sugar issues as the coconut oil helps slow down the impact of the carrots. A perfect drink for a "2 day" or any day!

5 large carrots
2 stalks of celery
1 cucumber
1 apple
Fresh ginger to taste
1 heaping T. coconut oil

1. Juice carrots, celery, cucumber and apple.
2. Pour into blender.
3. Add ginger and coconut oil and blend on high.

Makes approximately 2 servings of juice.

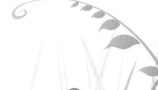

Kidney Tonic

A fabulous juice to help purify and support the kidneys. This juice is a diuretic and has wonderful balancing minerals.

> 2 carrots
> 2 stalks celery
> 2 large beets with tops
> 1 large cucumber with skin
> 10 spinach leaves

Pour in a tall glass and stir in 1 tsp. barley grass powder (see *Get Equipped*).

Potassium-Packed Juice

This juice is fantastic for cleansing, alkalinizing, and rebuilding. Think of this juice as cell food.

> 3 carrots
> 1 small bunch of parsley
> 4 stalks of celery
> 1 bunch of fresh spinach
> 1 parsnip
> Beet greens (4 top leaves from beets thoroughly washed)
> 2 leaves of red leaf lettuce (optional)
> ¼ small green cabbage
> 1 red bell pepper
> 1 green apple (apples are the only fruit that can be juiced with veggies)

Makes approximately 2 servings of juice.

Wheatgrass Cocktail

Even if you don't like wheatgrass you are going to like this! Refreshing, tangy, and oh so cellularly healthy and vital!

> 1 oz. fresh wheatgrass
> Juice of one small lemon
> 2 apples, juiced

Mix all the juices together. Serves 1.

Cheers!

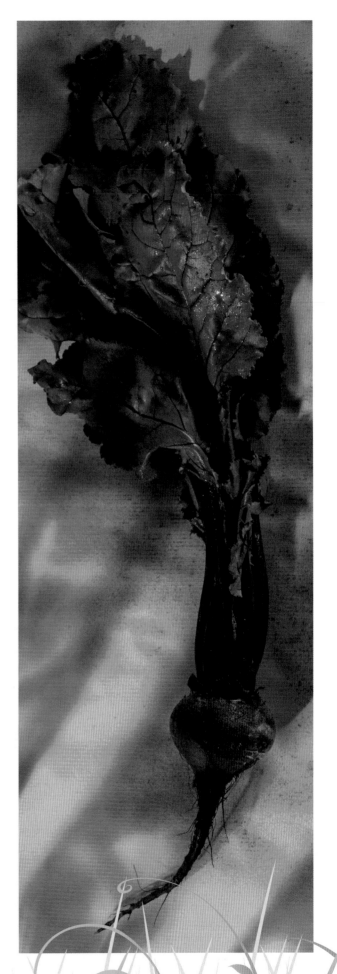

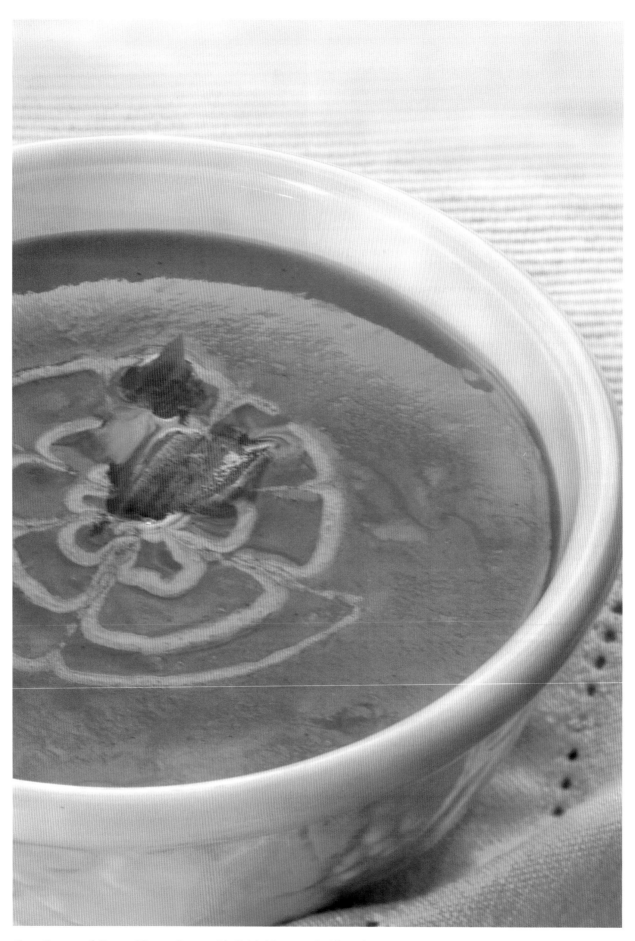

Raw Cream of Carrot Ginger Soup with Tahini Lemon Swirl, recipe on page 114.

Healing and Nourishing Broths and Soups

When I was so very sick after being poisoned, I remember one of those transforming intuitive times when I was laying in my bed with a sharp unrelenting pain in my left side. What it was I never knew, but what seemed to cure it came from the intuition I got to make and drink Bieler's Broth.

Dr. Bieler was best known for his best selling book *Food Is Your Best Medicine*. Respected as one of the pioneers of alternative medicine, he was quite successful using food instead of drugs and became popular with many celebrities including Greta Garbo, Lucille Ball, Anthony Quinn, and Gloria Swanson.

Although he died in 1975 at age 82, his legacy lives on and he fast became one of my heroes! I will never forget what a difference his original healing broth made for me!

Bieler's Broth

Great for detox and adrenal healing

4 med. courgettes (zucchini, yellow or summer)
1 lb. string beans, ends removed
2 stalks celery
2 bunches parsley, stems removed
Fresh herbs, such as thyme or tarragon, tied together with a string.
1 quart filtered water
Fresh whey, not powdered!! (optional)

Dr. Bieler recommended this broth for fasting, for energy, and overall health. He found this particular combination of vegetables was ideal for restoring acid-alkaline and sodium-potassium balance to organs and glands, especially the adrenal glands. Bieler broth is highly recommended for those under stress or suffering from stress-related conditions.

Place water, vegetables, and herbs in pot. Bring to a boil, then lower heat and simmer, covered for about ½ hour. Remove herbs. Eat as is or blend.

If you're a garlic lover, be sure to add some garlic and add Himalayan salt to taste. You may add 1 T. whey to each cup of broth or soup. Allow the soup to cool a bit before adding the whey so the heat does not damage the enzymes.

Homemade Whey

Why Whey? *(Shared by Paula at WholeIntentions.com)* Whey has been used for centuries. Icelanders preserved their food with whey, and Greek doctors referred to it as 'healing water.' Until the 1940's, spas in Europe treated gout, anemia, arthritis, and even tuberculosis with it. What did they know that we don't?

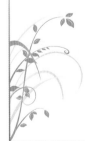 Whey is a protein that provides your body with an excellent source of minerals, essential amino acids, and digestive bacteria. In 2000, a study by the Arkansas Children's Nutrition Center found that whey may also prevent breast cancer.

Homemade Whey is Better. Many health food stores rightly tout the benefits of whey protein. But if you're really looking to build muscle, maintain your blood sugar, and boost your metabolism, skip the huge containers of powdered whey protein on the shelf and look no further than your own refrigerator.

Those powdered mixes contain artificial sweeteners, come from unknown sources (e.g. grain-fed, hormonally treated cows), they've obviously been processed in some way, and many of them contain heavy metals. Isn't that kind of counterproductive? To learn how to make whey, go to **www.WholeIntentions.com**.

Potassium Flush Broth

This is an excellent source of minerals and electrolytes. This broth is designed to help you flush out toxins and nourish your cells.

Place the following food list in a soup pot and then cover with water (at least 8 cups) and simmer with the lid on for 60 minutes. Strain and discard the veggies.

    4 carrots
    4 courgettes (zucchinis)
    1–2 leeks
    4 stalks celery
    1 head purple cabbage
    1 bunch kale
    1 bunch collards or chard
      bay leaves
    3 potatoes, scrubbed with skins
    1 onion
    6 cloves garlic
    1 bunch of parsley
    1 bunch of broccoli
    2 pieces of kombu seaweed
    Sprig of fresh thyme

Sip on this broth throughout the day. Let this replace your coffee! Store the broth in a large Mason jar with the lid on tight in the fridge and warm up as you need.

OPTIONS: For more nutrients and flavor, you can stir in whey or a small amount of miso paste into your soup bowl/cup. Non-vegans can add poultry bones for great added nutritional value.

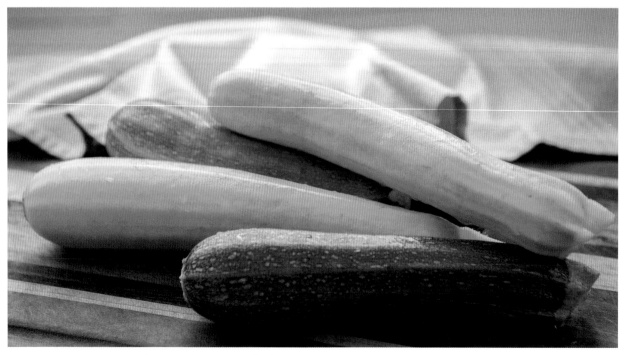

Known as courgettes in the UK, these are called zucchini in the US.

Homemade Vegetable Stock

This can be a stock used as a base for soups or it can be a potassium broth to sip on during "2 days."

Throw in any amounts of the following (and anything else hanging around your refrigerator), skins and all, as long as everything is thoroughly washed:

Purple cabbage
Courgettes (zucchini)
Parsnips
Swedes (optional)
String beans
Celery
Potatoes
Bunch of parsley
Bunch of coriander (cilantro)
Kale
Leeks
Beets
2 or 3 strips of kombu seaweed
12 whole cloves of garlic
Garlic salt
Himalayan salt to taste
Cayenne pepper to taste
Fresh ginger (optional)

1. Fill stockpot half full with water. Boil, then throw in veggies.
2. Turn down heat and let simmer about one hour.
3. Pour through a strainer and discard veggies. More than likely you will have a very pretty, purple, nourishing mineral broth/stock.

Vegetable Curry Soup

4 onions chopped
3 cloves garlic chopped
turmeric – a thumb-sized piece, finely chopped
1 red bell pepper, chopped
3 large carrots, finely sliced
1–2 T. butter
2 tsp. curry powder
1 tsp. garam masala
3 pods cardamom, crushed and use the seeds inside
¼ teaspoon hot red chili flakes
A few grinds of black pepper

1. Sauté above ingredients for 5–10 minutes until onions and carrots soften.
2. Add vegetable or bone broth (or 3 pints water). Bring to boil.
3. Add:
   3 yams, cubed
   1 potato, cubed
   ½–1 pound fresh mushrooms, sliced
   2 zucchinis, sliced
   1 pumpkin, peeled, cleaned of seeds and cubed
   ½ cup dry lentils
   ¼ pound chopped broccoli, cauliflower or romanesco
4. Let simmer for 60 to 90 minutes. Add Himalayan salt if desired.
5. Once soup has cooled a bit, serve with whole plain goat yogurt and/or whey.

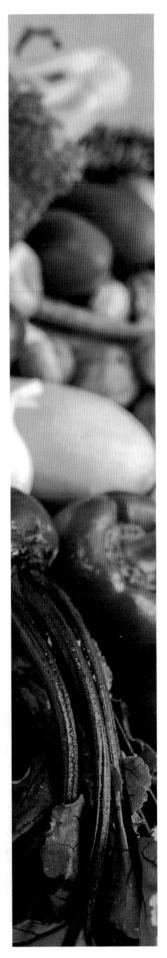

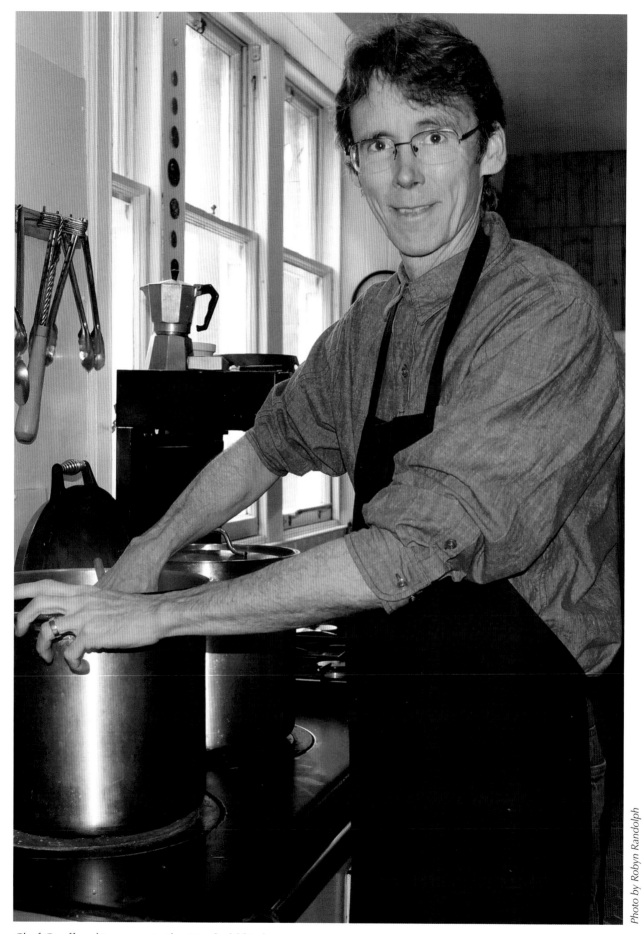

Chef Geoff making soup in the Newbold kitchen.

Photo by Robyn Randolph

Oat Groats and Shiitake Mushroom Soup

This is a very satisfying soup for a chilly day. I love to use shiitakes as they are an amazing super food containing eighteen amino acids, B vitamins, and a polysaccharide known as lentinan, which increases T-cell function, strengthening the immune system.

>   1 red onion, diced
>   2 T. olive oil or organic butter
>   8 cups organic vegetable broth
>   1 cup fresh shiitake mushrooms, sliced
>   3 cups oat groats, (gluten free as long as it is grown separate from wheat and barley)
>   2 carrots, grated

1. Heat oil or melt butter in a large soup pot. Sauté onions and mushrooms covered for 5 minutes.

2. Add the broth, oat groats and seasonings to taste and simmer for about 40 minutes over low heat.

3. Stir in the grated carrots at the end and enjoy!

Blended Winter Warming Soup

>   4 T. organic butter
>   1 yellow onion, chopped
>   1 red onion, chopped
>   2 leeks
>   1 T. fresh ginger, chopped
>   1 T. turmeric
>   2 red bell peppers, chopped
>   1 celeriac chopped
>   1 bunch of celery chopped
>   6 large carrots chopped
>   2 large butternut squashes—peel and split open, then scrape out seeds
>   4 yams peeled and chopped
>   2 cups dried yellow split peas
>   ½ tsp. cayenne
>   1 tsp. cumin seeds in the sauté
>   1 T. powdered cumin
>   1 tsp. cardamom
>   Himalayan salt
>   Vegetable broth/stock, bone broth or water to cover

1. Sauté onions, leeks, red bell peppers, celeriac, ginger, cumin seeds and turmeric in butter until onions are soft (add a little water if need be).

2. Add remaining ingredients with enough broth/water to cover and bring to a boil.

3. Reduce heat and simmer 1.5 hours.

4. Blend the soup into a puree.

Raw Enzyme Energy Soup

This soup is made completely in a blender. With a powerful motor such as the Enpee Blender or Vitamix, just two or three cycles on high will warm the soup up (but not hot enough to destroy the enzymes).

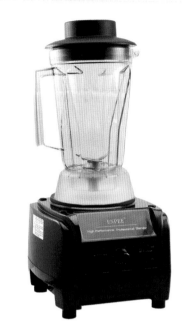

2 whole tomatoes, quartered
1 red bell pepper, cut in chunks
1 cucumber, cut into small chunks
Handful of kale, collards, or spinach
1 courgette (zucchini)
2 carrots, cut into thirds
¼ – ½ avocado
4 green olives
fresh jalapeno to taste
1 clove garlic
1 tsp. white mellow miso
1 tsp. cumin
3 pitted dates
Handful of fresh coriander (cilantro)
Himalayan salt to taste

1. Blend all ingredients in a heavy-duty blender such as the Enpee Blender.
2. Top with red peppers and mushrooms diced small.

Raw Cream of Fresh Tomato Soup

4 large vine ripe tomatoes
4 fresh basil leaves
½ tsp. Himalayan salt
½ – 1 large ripe avocado

UK only: Looks and performs just like a Vita-Mix, but has a stronger motor and costs over £200 less! Available at: **www.purehighlandliving. com/shop/blending**

Photo courtesy of Enpee Enterprises Ltd

Blend all ingredients in heavy-duty blender such as the Enpee or Vitamix. This is especially delicious when tomatoes are at the peak of the season.

OPTION: Add 1 tsp. Walnut Pesto (recipe on page 121) per bowl of soup.

Raw Cream of Carrot Ginger Soup with Tahini Lemon Swirl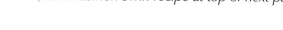

See photo of this dish on page 114.

¼ cup raw cashews (more if you want it thicker)
1 small tomato
1 T. fresh grated ginger (more if you like)
1 T. lemon juice
1 cup water (or more)
6 – 8 carrots
1 red bell pepper
1 tsp. coconut oil (optional)
½ avocado (optional as a thickener)
Himalayan salt to taste

1. Grind up the cashews into a powder first. Then add water and blend.
2. Add all other ingredients. Blend until smooth and long enough to get the motor hot enough to warm up the soup. *NOTE:* This requires a high-powered blender.

(Tahini Lemon Swirl recipe at top of next page)

Tahini Lemon Swirl

¼ cup tahini
2 T. lemon juice
Himalayan salt to taste
Coconut water as needed to thin out the sauce

1. Combine all ingredients and mix until smooth, the consistency is that of a thick oil. Add coconut water if needed. (The personal blender is great for this.)

2. Using a bottle with a narrow cap (such as a mustard bottle) or an eyedropper, drizzle the swirl sauce however you want on the top of the soup. This makes for a festive and visually appetizing soup.

Minted Courgette and Pea Soup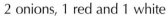

2 onions, 1 red and 1 white
3 T. butter
2 leeks, chopped
3 large courgettes, chopped
4 apples, chopped
1–2 cups vegetable broth or chicken stock
A huge handful of spinach
A generous handful of fresh mint
A small package of organic frozen peas
Himalayan salt and pepper
Garlic salt

1. In a soup pot, sauté the red and yellow onions in butter.

2. Add chopped leeks and sauté until soft.

3. Add all other ingredients except for frozen peas.

4. Simmer until everything is soft and ready for blending.

5. Use a hand blender right in the pot or liquefy in blender.

6. Pour back into pot and warm up, adding frozen peas.

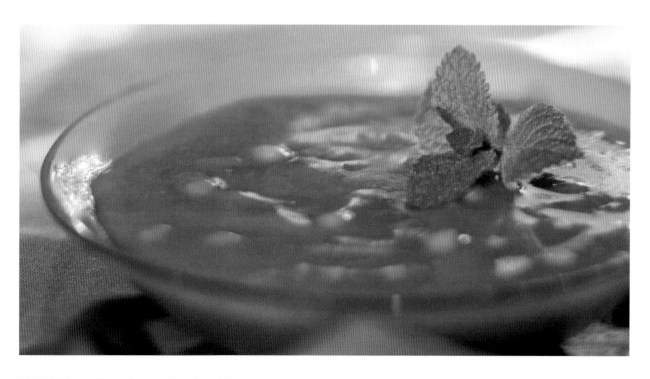

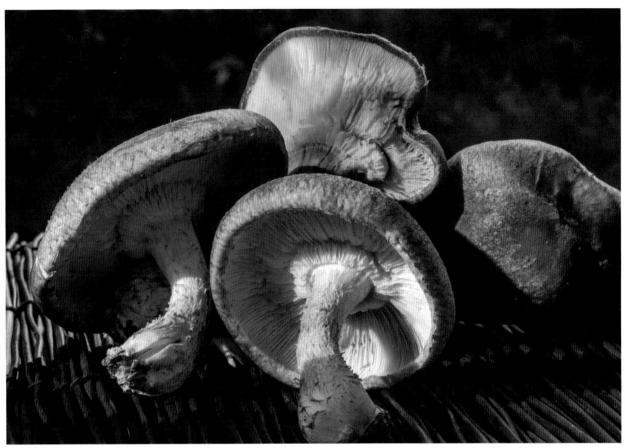

A powerful antioxidant, the Chinese have used shiitake mushrooms for medicinal purposes for over 6,000 years.

Shiitake Soul Soup

Shiitakes are known for their high therapeutic value. Think of this soup when you want to boost your immune system. Subtle but extremely nourishing to every cell, this is a perfect flu season soup. This is one of those "...let food be your medicine" soups!

    1 ounce dried shiitake mushrooms
    1 long piece of kombu (Japanese dried kelp), cut into small pieces
    12 fresh shiitake mushrooms sliced thin
    Bunch of fresh chives, diced fine
    3 T. nama shoyu
    1 tsp. honey
    ½ tsp. toasted sesame oil
    3 drops brown rice vinegar
    2-inch piece of burdock root (optional)
    Lemongrass stalk

1. In a soup pot, soak the dried mushrooms in 6 cups of hot water for half an hour.

2. Using kitchen scissors cut the kombu into small pieces and add to the pot.

3. For a more therapeutic soup, add the burdock root now, bring to boil, reduce heat and simmer for 5 minutes.

4. Strain the stock. Press firmly to extract as much liquid as possible. Add the fresh shiitake mushrooms and ¾ of the chives.

5. In a small bowl mix together the honey, sesame oil, and vinegar. Mix into soup pot.
   Cut lemongrass stalk with kitchen scissors and add to soup.

6. Cook soup over medium heat, covered, until the mushrooms are tender, about 30 minutes.

7. Serve in bowls and garnish with the remaining chives.

RawSome Ratatouille

I designed this soup to be hearty, warming and still include the enzymatic benefits of some uncooked foods. Using raw grated carrots, diced avocados and sunflower sprouts to top off the bowl adds flare, fresh flavor and enzymes.

Home Base Sauce (see page 119)
1 large red onion and 1 large white onion
1 large eggplant, cubed (remove skin if you wish)
2 large zucchinis, sliced
2 large yellow squash
2 large red bell peppers
1 large can of organic chopped tomatoes

3 cups broth or purified water (less if you want it to be thicker)
Handful of whole peeled cloves of garlic
1 tsp. garlic powder
1 tsp. onion powder
1 tsp. Italian seasoning
1 tsp. cinnamon

Use as much or as little as you wish of the following:

Garbanzo beans (better would be fresh home-cooked garbanzo, and best would be sprouted*)
Avocados
Sunflower sprouts (or any sprouts available)
Grated carrots
Currants (optional)

1. In a large stockpot pour enough Home Base Sauce to cover bottom of pot. Sauté onions until soft and translucent.

2. Add zucchinis, peppers, tomatoes, eggplant, whole cloves of garlic, seasonings and water or broth (for more of a stew add less water or broth).

3. Cook until all ingredients are soft but not mushy. Add garbanzo beans and mix all ingredients together.

4. Top with fresh grated carrots, diced avocado, and sunflower sprouts.

*OPTION: To enhance this dish with wonderful enzymes, think ahead three days. Soak one cup dried garbanzo beans in water for two hours. Then sprout for three full days, remembering to rinse well, 2–4 times throughout the day. Wait until Ratatouille has cooled down, so as to not destroy the valuable enzymes, and then mix in the sprouted garbanzo beans. This can be served over cooked oat groats or quinoa.

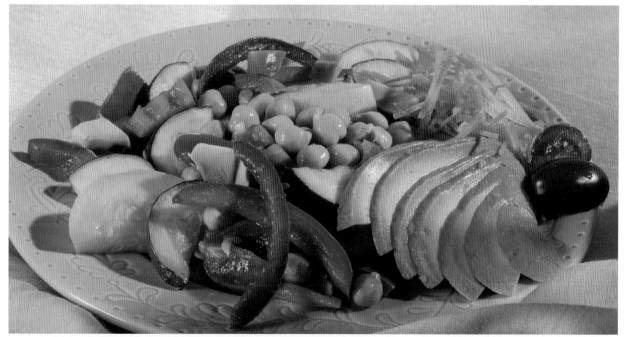

When making this recipe, you can set aside some of the ingredients for a wonderful raw snack. A great way to sneak in a little extra raw food during your day!

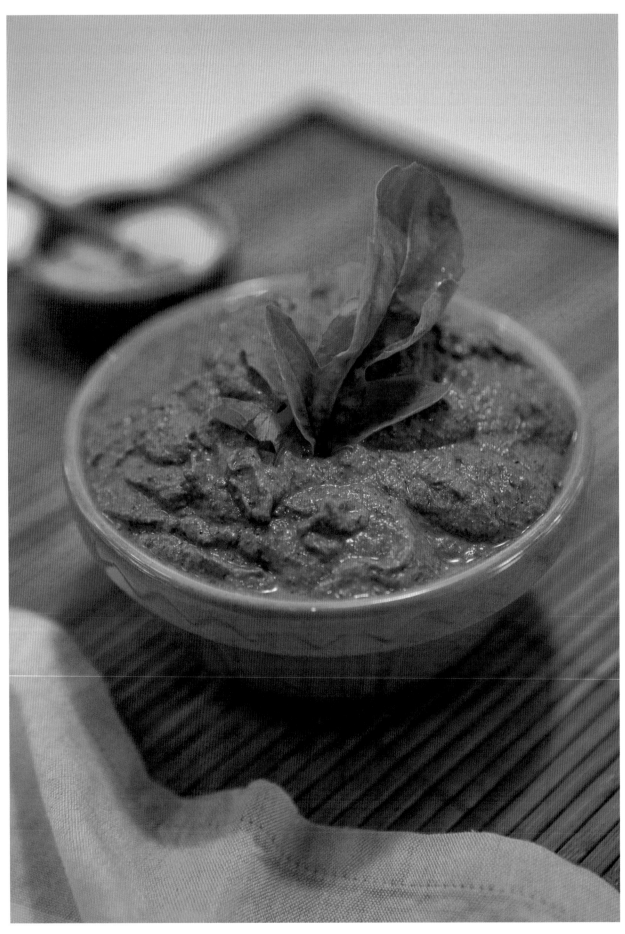

Walnut Pesto Sauce, recipe on page 121.

PURE Salad Dressings, Sauces and Condiments:

Home Base Sauce & House Dressing

I call this dressing Home Base Sauce because I use it in multiple recipes. It is a great marinade, salad dressing, and base for sautéing onions, mushrooms, or veggies. It is helpful to keep a jar of this ready-to-go, in the fridge!

> 1 cup organic olive oil
> Juice of 2 lemons (Meyer lemons are the best)
> 6–8 cloves garlic minced
> 2 T. fruit juice sweetened apricot jam
> 1 tsp. cumin
> 1 tsp. Italian seasoning
> Himalayan salt to taste

Place all ingredients in a canning jar, making sure lid is tight, and shake vigorously.

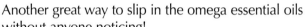

Honey Mustard a la Udo's

Another great way to slip in the omega essential oils without anyone noticing!

> 2 T. Udo's Oil
> Juice of 1 lemon
> 1–2 tsp. stone ground salt-free mustard
> 1 tsp. manuka honey

Mix all ingredients in blender. Adjust to taste by adding more honey.

We love using the Tribest Personal Blender to make salad dressings.

Creamy Garlic

This is another great dressing to blend up and store in a sealed jar in the fridge, ready to go when you are ready to use it! Also great as a dip with sliced raw kohlrabies.

> 2 T. "Honegar" (a UK product that combines honey and apple cider vinegar)
> ¼ cup olive oil or grape seed oil (for a lighter flavor)
> 1–2 cloves garlic
> date syrup to taste
> goat yogurt (optional)
> 1 T. soaked cashews (optional)

Poppy Seed Lime Salad Dressing

> Juice of 1 or 2 limes
> ¼ cup Udo's Oil or olive oil
> 1 tsp. poppy seeds
> 1 tsp. honey or 1–2 pitted medjool dates
> Himalayan salt to taste

Blend all ingredients except poppy seeds (stir in at the end).

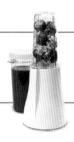

Ginger Sesame Dressing

4 T. olive and/or Udo's Oil
2 T. brown rice vinegar
1 tsp. fresh grated ginger
1½ T. raw honey
1 T. sesame seeds
1 clove garlic, minced to taste
Himalayan salt to taste

Blend and serve.

Red Bell Pepper & Almond Dressing

1 cup almonds, soaked overnight,
   then rinsed and drained
1 red bell pepper
1 cup purified water
   (more if needed as it thickens in time)
1 or 2 garlic cloves
1 tsp. nutritional yeast
2 pitted dates

Add Udo's oil if you like. Mix ingredients in blender.

Sweet Curry Dressing

4 T. olive oil
1 T. Udo's Oil (optional)
2 T. fresh lemon juice
2 cloves garlic
1 tsp. curry powder
½ tsp. cumin
½ tsp. powdered ginger or
   1 tsp. fresh ginger
4 pitted dates, soaked until soft
Himalayan salt to taste
1 tsp. honey (more if you like)

Blend in blender and add cashews if you want it creamier.

Red Head Dressing

¼ cup olive oil
2 ripe tomatoes
½ red bell pepper
1 T. brown rice vinegar
1 tsp. apricot jam or 1–2 pitted dates
1–2 cloves garlic

Blend all ingredients. Great served on red leaf lettuce!

Green Goodness Dressing

½ cup lemon juice
½ cup olive oil
1 slice fresh ginger
1 clove garlic
1 heaping T. Tahini
1 T. honey (can add more or less)
1 bunch fresh cilantro
½ bunch fresh parsley
Himalayan salt to taste

Blend and serve.

Ginger Yum Yum Sauce

½ cup of each of the following:
   Fresh lemon juice
   Raw tahini butter
   Maple syrup or date syrup
   Wheat-free soy sauce (tamari)
2 cloves garlic, diced small
½ –1 tsp. fresh ginger, grated
   (or more if you love ginger!)

Mix everything together in the blender and store in a glass jar in the fridge.

OPTIONS: You can also use this recipe as a dip with fresh cut-up veggies as a starter. I like to add fresh cilantro, parsley and/or mint to the above ingredients. The fresh herbs add a dimension to the sauce, transforming it into a great salad dressing.

PURE Immune Boost Salad Dressing or Tincture

Make this salad dressing and have it on hand for the cold/flu season. Use it as a daily tonic: on salads and lettuce wraps, to perk up soups, dips, stir fries, steamed vegetables, in vegetable juices or as a tincture by the dropperful!

- ½ cup raw apple cider vinegar
- 3 garlic cloves
- 1 inch of fresh ginger (or more to taste)
- Generous pinch of Himalayan salt and black pepper
- 1 tsp. tumeric powder, or a nice chunk if you are lucky enough to get it fresh
- 1½ cups organic extra virgin olive oil
- Jalepeno pepper (as much or as little as you can stand!)
- 1 T. manuka honey (or to taste)
- 1 T. mild miso paste
- Juice of one lime

Toss salad with a generous amount of dressing and for an added boost squeeze a fresh lime and toss again.

Eat well and be well! Cheers...

Walnut Pesto Sauce

The two tricks to making a great pesto are:

1. Be sure to remove the leaves and discard the stems of the basil, as the stems make it bitter.

2. Use the mildest and purest-tasting organic olive oil, making sure it does not have a bitter aftertaste.

Try stirring a big tablespoon of this pesto into soups like minestrone or garden vegetable to bring a vibrant dimension. Although you can certainly use the traditional pine nuts, we like to use walnuts for their great nutritional value including being a great omega fat.

First blend:

- ¾ cup organic olive oil
- 2–4 cloves minced garlic, depending on taste

Then add and blend together:

- 4 T. of walnuts (soaked for at least 1 hour)
- 1 large bunch of fresh basil
- 2 tsp. apricot jam or 2–4 soft pitted dates
- 1–2 T. lemon juice
- Himalayan salt to taste
- Pinch of paprika

Raw Marinara Sauce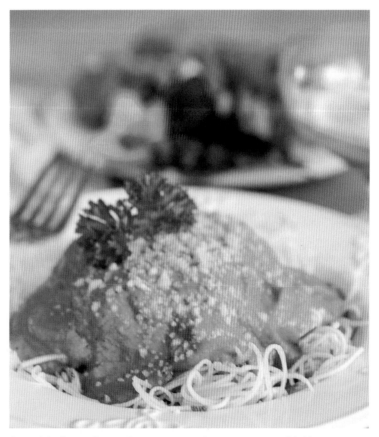

- 3 cups of blended tomatoes
- A couple handfuls of sundried tomatoes (about 2 cups), soaked for 2 hours, or use jarred, oil-soaked tomatoes
- 2 T. fruit juice-sweetened apricot jam, or 2–4 pitted soft dates
- 1 T. Italian seasoning
- 1–2 cloves of fresh garlic
- ½ sweet onion
- 4 leaves of fresh basil
- 2 T. fresh parsley
- Touch of olive oil
- 2 T. capers
- Himalayan salt to taste
- Black olives (optional)

Blend all together in a high-speed blender.

Raw Marinara Sauce is great served over raw zucchini/courgette angel hair pasta, made with a spiralizer. Finely grind macadamia nuts for mock parmesan cheese!

Macadamia Mayonnaise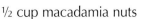

½ cup macadamia nuts
½ cup cashews
¼ cup lemon juice
½ clove garlic
¼ cup coconut water
Himalayan salt to taste

OPTION: Add ⅛ tsp. Dijon mustard and/or ⅛ tsp. honey apple cider vinegar.

Blend all ingredients until smooth and creamy. Adjust coconut water for desired consistency. Store in glass jar in the fridge.

Sour Cashew Cream

Use this recipe in place of sour cream. Great for Mexican dishes!

1 cup raw cashews, soaked for at least 2 hours, then drained)
½ cup water
¼ cup lemon juice
1 tsp. apple cider vinegar
¼ tsp. Himalayan salt
1 T. fresh liquid whey (optional)

Blend everything in the blender until completely smooth. Chill and enjoy! Good for up to a week in the fridge.

NOTE: Add more or less water for desired consistency.

Spicy BBQ Ketchup

This delicious sauce is great for making kale and courgettes chips. Just marinate and pop in the dehydrator. Use in place of store-bought ketchup. Leave out the jalepenos if you like it mild.

1 cup fresh tomatoes, chopped
½ cup sun dried tomatoes, (packed in olive oil)
¼ jalepeno or more if you like it HOT
¾ cup pitted, soft dates
½ cup sweet or yellow onion
½ tsp. minced fresh garlic
1 tsp. Himalayan salt
4 fresh basil leaves
Olive oil for blending (can use oil in the jar from sundried tomatoes)
Red pepper flakes (as much or as little as you like)
1 tsp. mesquite seasoning or Cajun spice
Pinch or two of smoked paprika

Blend all together until smooth in high speed blender.

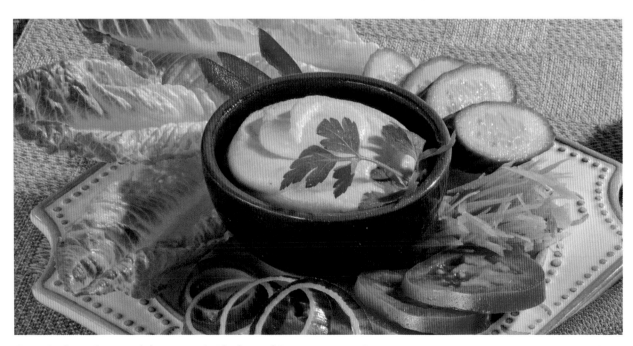

Sour Cashew Cream, delicious with Black-eyed Peas & Lettuce Burritos, recipe on page 122.

PURE Cranberry Relish:

This tangy citrus relish is a perfect holiday-time condiment. I recommend trying this with the pomegranate seeds, as they create an unusual texture and add a surprise flavor twist.

    2 cups fresh or frozen cranberries
    ¼ small red onion
    6 pitted dates
    2 tsp. fresh grated ginger
    2 T. lemon juice
    Zest of ½ orange
    ½ cup grated carrot
    2 tangerines, sectioned and cut up into small pieces
    Himalayan salt to taste
    Pomegranate seeds (optional)

1. Place cranberries and onion in processor and pulse chop. Put in a bowl.

2. Process dates, lemon juice, ginger, salt and orange zest. Pulse in the shredded carrots.

3. Add the two mixtures. Pulse in the pomegranate seeds if you like the taste and coarse texture that pomegranates create.

4. Fold in the tangerines.

5. Refrigerate overnight to blend the flavors. Will keep in the refrigerator for about 10 days.

OPTION: Add ½ cup fresh cilantro, ½ jalepeno diced for a little zip, some chopped walnuts and/or currants. Any and all of these are great additions.

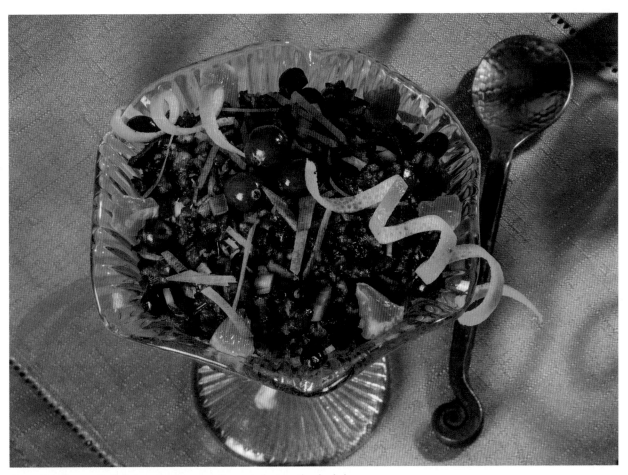

Pure Cranberry Relish is a festive condiment during the holiday season.

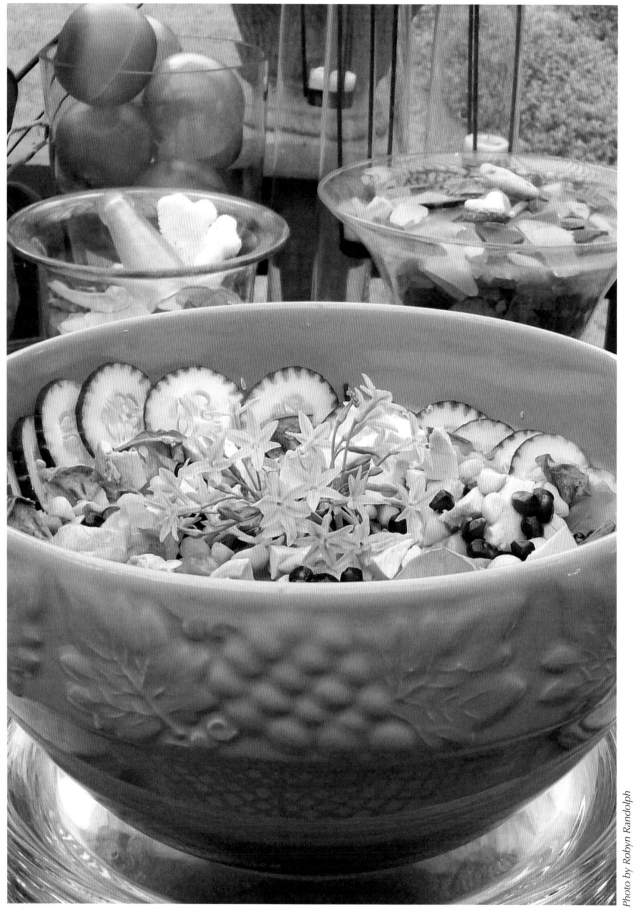

Salads can be as festive and as creative as you like. In this salad I used dried persimmons and pomegranite seeds for a lovely high anitoxidant boost.

PURE Salads

As an "intuitive chef" I love to work with whatever presents itself in the moment. For me, food is living art and I like to use edible flowers to create my salad masterpieces!

Yellow & Red Cherry Tomato Salad

Tomatoes with basil and garlic… always a winning combination!

White sweet corn kernels from 2 ears
2 cups of assorted sweet yellow and red cherry tomatoes
½ red onion, diced
½ cup basil, cut into small pieces
2 – 3 cloves garlic minced fine
½ cup fresh lemon juice
3 T. olive oil
Himalayan salt to taste

1. Mix garlic, lemon juice, oil, kelp and salt (to taste) in a nice serving bowl.

2. Slice tomatoes in half and then add with remaining ingredients into bowl.

3. Toss and serve on individual salad plates. Serves 2 – 4.

Spa Salad

1 large head of butter lettuce
2 small apples, cut in small chunks
Fresh fennel, sliced like celery pieces
1 large avocado, sliced
1 red bell pepper, sliced in strips
Pecans or walnuts

1. Toss lettuce, apples, and fennel in a large serving bowl or platter with Home Base Dressing (see page 119).

2. Fan out the avocado slices into a circle on top, in the center of the salad.

3. Sprinkle nuts to top the salad.

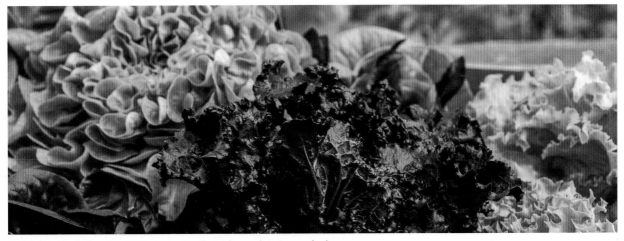

Fresh-picked organic lettuce is the best base for any salad.

Kale Salad with Ginger Yum Yum Sauce

This is my favorite kale recipe and everyone always seems to love it. Even kids, which says a lot. You'll find Ginger Yum Yum Sauce recipe on page 120.

Use as much or as little as you like of the following ingredients:

  2 bunches of kale, washed,
    spun dry, cut in small pieces
  ¼ – ½ small purple cabbage diced
    into very small pieces
  ½ cup currants (or more)
  ½ – 1 cup soaked and sprouted
    sunflower seeds

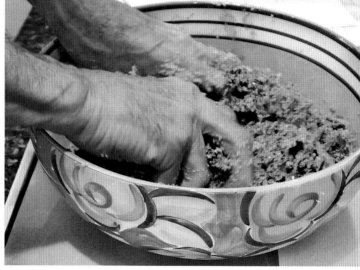

1. Soak sunflower seeds for two hours.
2. Using a mesh strainer, pour off the water, give them a rinse and let them sprout in a sunny spot for 1 day.
3. Place all ingredients into a large mixing bowl.
4. Pour enough Ginger Yum Yum Sauce to coat kale leaves well.
5. Roll up your sleeves, and with clean hands, massage the sauce

Massaging the kale salad at a PURE 5:2 workshop.

into the kale. Toss and massage everything well, which helps to break down the kale.
6. Let stand at room temperature to marinate for 1 – 6 hours before serving.

Christmas Kale Salad

This is a jazzed-up version of Kale Salad with Ginger Yum Yum Sauce (above). I use a spiral slicer to get my beets to come out looking like this. Start with the above ingredients, and add:

  Fresh red currants
  2 persimmons, sliced and then sliced again in half to create a half-moon shape
  1 large red beet (sliced with a Saladaco Spiral Slicer)
  2 sliced figs

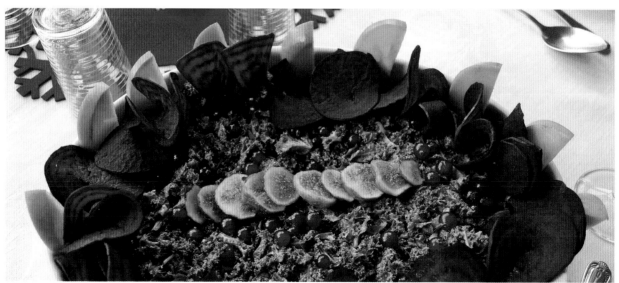

Using persimmons in this dish adds not only a great visual appeal but a great high antioxidant boost as well.

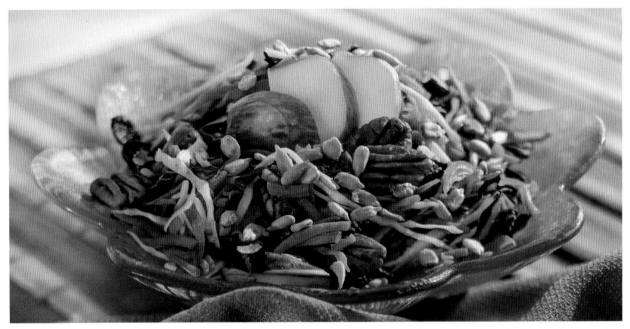

Sprouted sunflower seeds are rich in good fats, the water soluble B-complex vitamins, and vitamin E, as well as the metabolism-enhancing minerals copper, magnesium, and manganese.

Sprouted Sunflower Seed Salad

When the garden is quiet during winter, grow things indoors! Soak sunflower seeds in water to cover for 2 hours. Strain and rinse. Place near natural sunlight and let sprout in mesh strainer until tails appear! (A few hours or overnight.)

> 4 large carrots, grated
> ½ cup soaked sunflower seeds
> ¼ raw green and/or red cabbage, grated
> 1 apple, quartered and very thinly sliced
> 1 red bell pepper, halved, de-seeded and thinly sliced
> ¼ cup dried currants
> ¼ cut chopped pecans (can substitute walnuts)

6. Mix all ingredients together in a salad bowl.

7. Make up a batch of Creamy Garlic dressing (see page 119) and pour over salad and toss well.

8. Sprinkle sesame seeds on top. Add cracked pepper to taste.

4. Arrange sliced bell peppers around the outside edge of the bowl. Serves 2.

Purple Confetti Salad

> 1 large head of romaine lettuce
> 1 red onion, diced
> 4 celery stalks, diced small
> 1 red beet, shredded in food processor
> 4 ripe tomatoes, diced
> ½ cup sunflower seeds
> ½ small purple cabbage

1. Toss all ingredients with Honey Mustard a la Udo's Dressing (see page 119). Serve on large dinner plates. Use a paper towel to wipe the rim of the plate clean.

2. Turn cabbage into confetti with "S" blade of processor.

3. Sprinkle the purple confetti cabbage around the outside rim of the plate for a festive touch.

Serves 2–4.

Westernized Greek Salad with Capers

Adding capers and avocados to this salad takes it to a new dimension. I always make an extra large batch of this salad because we tend to make a meal out of it!

Organic feta cheese, for non-vegans. (It's best if you can find raw organic feta cheese.) Vegans can substitute with pieces of raw young coconut meat, if available.
1 red onion
3 cucumbers
12 pitted Kalamata olives, diced
½ jar of capers
4 cloves of garlic, minced
8 plump juicy ripe tomatoes
1 large avocado, diced
Himalayan salt to taste

Mix all the ingredients together and chill. Top with Creamy Garlic Dressing (page 119).

Popeye's Special Spinach Salad

2–4 cups tender young fresh spinach
4 or 5 ripe tomatoes, diced
½ red onion, diced
½–1 cup red kidney beans (optional)
Diced avocado

Assemble and toss with Honey Mustard Dressing a la Udo's (see page 119).

Non-vegan Option: Add two to four hard boiled eggs plus crumbled organic goat feta cheese.

Serves 2–4.

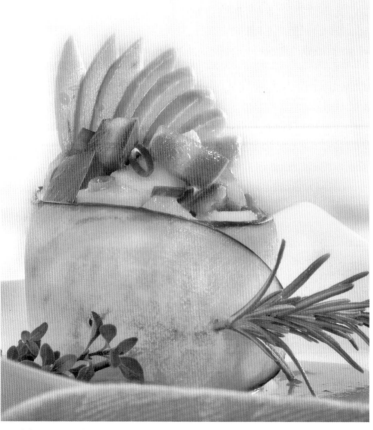

Building up salads, as shown in this picture, is visual eye candy for the person being served. We eat with our eyes.

Waldorf Salad with Macadamia Mayo

6–8 apples
Walnuts
Currants
Celery
Macadamia mayonnaise
(see page 122).

Use as much or as little of each ingredient and toss with macadamia mayonnaise.

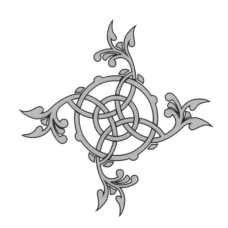

Asian Pear Salad with Mint Dressing

Warning: The mint dressing on this salad is highly addictive!

1 head romaine lettuce
    1 ripe avocado, diced
    1–2 Asian pears, diced
    ¼ small red onion, diced fine
    Handful of mixed nuts

Mint Dressing:

    juice of 1 lemon
    ½ cup olive oil
    1 clove garlic
    2 T. Udo's Oil or flax oil (optional)
    1 large bunch of fresh mint
    1 T. honey or maple syrup
    Himalayan salt to taste

1. Arrange salad in bowl using all the ingredients.

2. Toss with dressing and serve.

Serves 2–4. You can store leftover dressing in a glass jar with a lid in fridge for about a week.

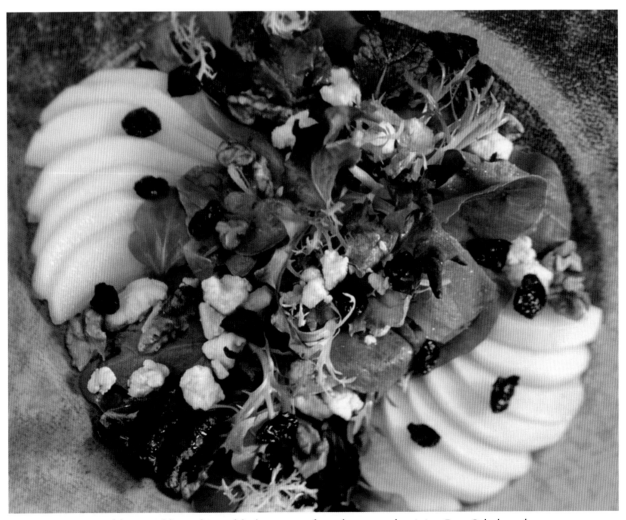

Non-vegans can add a sprinkling of crumbled raw goat feta cheese to the Asian Pear Salad, and vegans can substitute Creamed Mac Spread (recipe on page 133).

Marinated Green Beans & Walnuts in Apricot Dressing

1 lb. green beans, blanched
½ cup chopped fresh basil
1 small red onion, diced
2 stalks celery, diced fine
Cherry tomatoes, sliced in half
Fresh corn off the cob
¾ cup chopped walnuts

1. Blanch green beans by immersing them in boiling water for 30–60 seconds.
2. Marinate all ingredients in Home Base Sauce (see page 119) but add one additional heaping tsp. of apricot jam.

Pomegranate and Persimmon Salad

Use as much or as little as you like of the ingredients listed below. This is a fun, festive, and fancy salad. Be creative with how you plate this! Have fun with it! Great served with Mint Dressing (see recipe with Asian Pear Salad).

Butter lettuce and/or Romaine
Pomegranate seeds
Macadamia nuts
Avocados
Dried persimmons (or dried mangos)
Cucumbers
Edible flowers

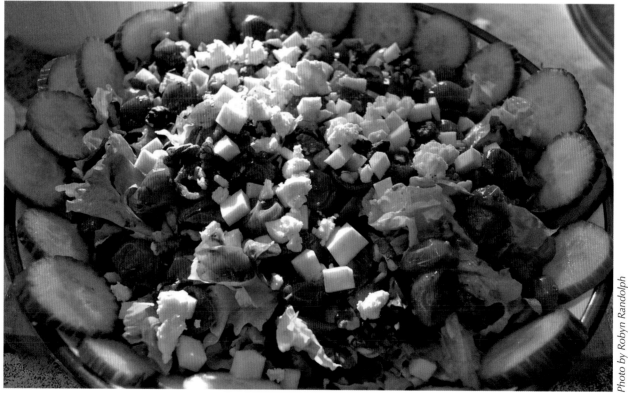

Take a fork and drag the prongs lengthwise from the top of the cucumber to the bottom. Repeat all the way around to get this pretty decorative look on your cuke slices.

Simple Salad for One

Start with the dressing:

1½ T. fresh lemon juice
1½ T. organic virgin olive oil
Himalayan salt to taste
1 clove garlic, minced
½ tsp. manuka honey

1. Place all ingredients above in the bottom of a medium-sized stainless steel salad bowl and stir vigorously, making sure the honey mixes in well.

2. Now add your favorite salad ingredients. It can be as simple as lettuce and tomatoes. I like to do lettuce, fresh chopped tomatoes, diced sweet red onions, grated carrots, cucumbers, celery and fresh garden peas.

3. Toss well and eat right out of the bowl!

East West Mix Salad Supreme

1 small green cabbage, shredded
1 head romaine, washed and cut up
Fresh (or frozen) peas
1 bunch green spring onions, diced
Chopped fresh cilantro
Slivered almonds

Mix salad and toss with the following dressing:

⅓ cup olive oil (or blend with sesame oil)
Juice of ½ large, fresh orange or tangerine
Approx. 1 T. brown rice vinegar
1 tsp. honey
1 T. black sesame seeds

Serves 2–4.

Spinach Salad with Cashews & Shiitakes

A great wintertime salad. The addition of the warm sautéed mushrooms and onions adds a nice sizzling touch!

4 cups fresh young spinach leaves, rinsed and drained
One small carton orange cherry tomatoes, sliced in half
Large handful of shiitake mushrooms, sliced
1 medium red onion, diced
Butter to coat pan
½–¾ cup cashews

1. Sauté mushrooms and onions in enough butter to coat pan.

2. Put spinach in bowl and toss salad with Red Bell Pepper and Almond Dressing (see page 120).

3. Add cashews, tomatoes and mushrooms and give another toss. Serves 2.

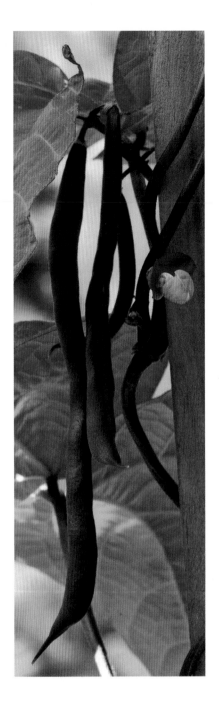

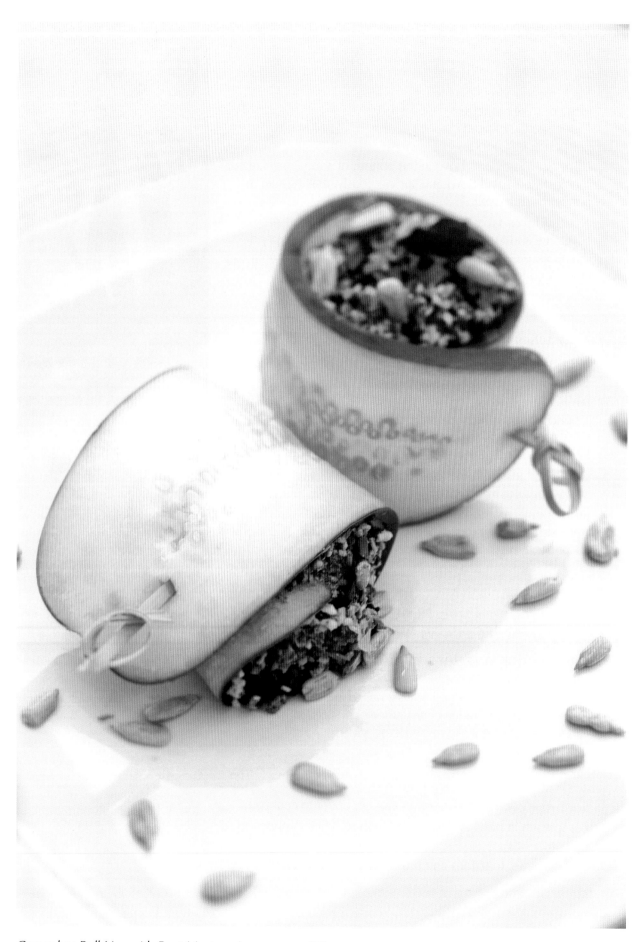

Cucumber Roll Ups with Beet Meat, recipe on page 138.

132

PURE Bites and Raw Dinner Delights:

Creamed Mac Spread on Cucumber Chips

1 cup macadamia nuts
½ cup cashews
½ cup lemon juice
1 T. minced garlic
1½ tsp. Himalayan salt
¼ – ½ cup water
Cucumbers
Chives
Cherry tomatoes, quartered
Smoked paprika

1. Grind nuts into flour using "S" blade in the processor.
2. Mix first six ingredients in food processor, adding water slowly to make a smooth spread.
3. Spread on cucumber rounds and top with chives and tomatoes.
4. Sprinkle with smoked paprika.

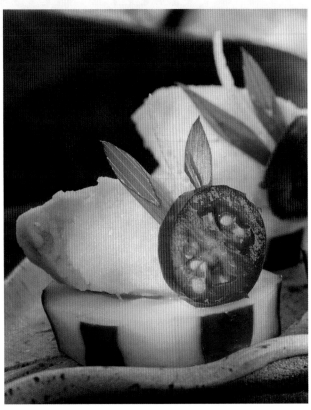

With their festive red and green colors, these make great Christmas season hors d'oeuvres!

Black-eyed Peas Lettuce Burritos

If you love the flavors of Mexico but don't love the grains that go with them, then this is the burrito for you!

1 cup black-eyed peas
Romaine lettuce leaves
1–2 avocados
Juice of ½ lemon
½ tsp. garlic powder
Himalayan salt to taste
8–10 pitted olives, diced
2 T. diced red onion
Organic salsa
Smoked paprika
Sour Cashew Cream (see page 122)

1. Cook peas in enough water to cover (soak and rinse first if you have time). These cook fairly quickly so keep an eye on them (approximately 20 minutes).
2. Blend avocado, lemon juice, garlic powder and salt to taste in blender (the personal blender works great for this). Drain peas and mix with onions.
3. Spoon pea mixture onto lettuce leaves, top with salsa, avocado, diced olives and Sour Cashew Cream. Dust with smoked paprika.

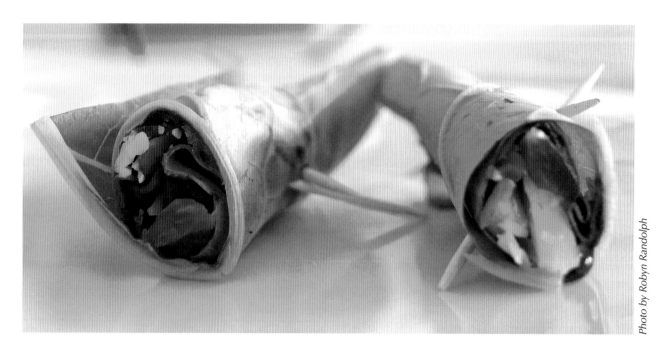

Kale Wraps

  1 large kale leaf
  ½ mejdool date
  ½ oz. sauerkraut, chopped
  3 walnut halves, chopped
  Lemon Garlic Hummus (see recipe below)

Place all ingredients on kale leaf and roll up. Contain with toothpicks.

Lemon Garlic Hummus

  1 can of garbanzo beans (chick peas), drained and rinsed
  ⅓ cup tahini
  juice from 1 large lemon
  pinch of freshly grated lemon rind
  ¼ cup water
  ⅓ cup extra virgin olive oil
  2 cloves fresh garlic
  1 tsp. Himalayan salt
  ½ tsp. asafoetida
  1 clove garlic
  Smoked paprika
  Sliced red, orange, and yellow bell peppers
  OPTION: Add in left over almond pulp from making almond milk

1. Place all ingredients except sliced peppers, in blender on medium speed and blend until creamy, smooth texture is achieved.

2. Adjust seasonings, if necessary. Garnish with smoked paprika and more olive oil. Serve with bell pepper slices.

Cashew Paté/Solar Tacos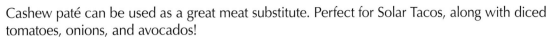

Cashew paté can be used as a great meat substitute. Perfect for Solar Tacos, along with diced tomatoes, onions, and avocados!

Paté:

>   1 cup cashews
>   1 cup sunflower seeds
>   1 jar organic salsa

1. Blend cashews and sunflower seeds in food processor into a fine powder.

2. Add salsa from the jar and blend into pate or "taco meat."

Solar Tacos:

>   Cashew Paté
>   Fresh salsa
>   Avocado
>   Diced tomatoes
>   Chopped onion
>   Romaine lettuce leaves

3. Use lettuce leaves for the taco shell and scoop the nut/seed "meat" into the middle.

4. Top with fresh salsa, avocado, diced tomatoes, and onions.

OPTION: Instead of lettuce leaves, use Carrot Tortillas (see page 137)!

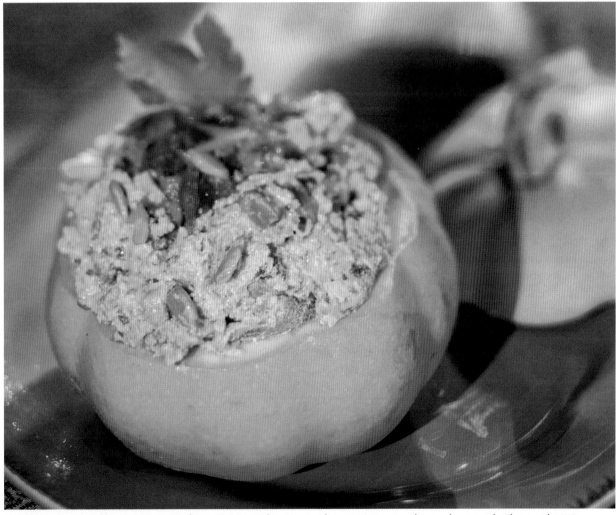

In the autumn, I like to serve Cashew Paté inside scooped-out mini pumpkins, along with Flax to the Max Crackers (recipe page 136)!

Flax To The Max Crackers

2 cups flax seeds, soaked 2 hours

1½ cups almonds, soaked 6–12 hours

2 cups carrot pulp or finely grated carrots
(approximately 4 large carrots)

1 medium red bell pepper, sliced into quarters
(ready for the processor)

½ red onion or sweet onion

½ cup fresh cilantro/coriander

3 T. olive oil

4 pitted dates, soaked for at least an hour first

2 T. fresh lemon juice

2 cloves garlic

1–2 tsp. curry powder

½ tsp. cumin

¼ tsp. turmeric

½–1 tsp. ginger powder

1½ tsp. Himalayan salt

1 tsp. red pepper flakes

1 tsp. honey

1. Grate carrots and grind almonds in a food processor. Transfer processed carrots and almonds into a bowl. *OPTIONS:* use leftover pulp from making carrot juice or almond milk, or put carrots and almonds through a juicer using the blank plate.

2. Mix oil and garlic in food processor.

3. Add lemon juice, honey and all spices. For more kick add more spices, especially the curry and red pepper flakes and blend until integrated.

4. Add the dates and continue to blend until mixture becomes a moist paste.

5. Continue by adding the onion and bell peppers.

6. Add the carrot and almond pulp into the processor and blend everything together.

7. Place the contents of the processor back into the large bowl and finally add the soaked flaxseeds. (They will have absorbed all the water and become quite gelatinous.) Use your hands to mix everything together well.

8. Using a spatula, spread cracker batter on drying sheet approximately ¼ inch thick.

9. Score crackers with tip of spatula and dehydrate at 47°/118°F for 6–8 hours.

10. Turn crackers over following steps shown at right.

11. Continue dehydrating for another 12–24 hours until crackers are very crisp.

Makes anywhere from 2–2½ trays of crackers.

Store in glass jars.

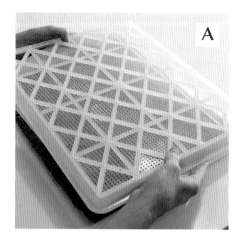

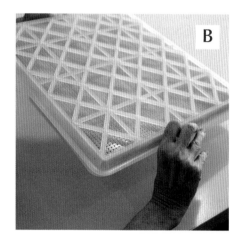

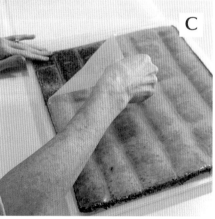

Photos by Geoff Randolph

Turning Over a Tray of Crackers

A. *Remove tray from dehydrator and place another tray over it upside down, with a screen only (no drying sheet).*

B. *Flip everything over and remove original tray.*

C. *Carefully peel away the drying sheet as you press the crackers into place on the screen-only tray.*

Chili Lime Carrot Tortillas, Wraps or Crackers

It will take a bit of effort and a few steps to create these delicious corn/wheat alternatives. However, let me assure you, it is well worth it as having raw tortillas, wraps, and crackers opens up a whole new dimension for raw food satisfaction and delight!

2¾ cups grated carrots or carrot pulp
½ cup pine nuts
½ cup coconut flour
2 yellow or red bell peppers
1 cup golden linseed/flaxseed, finely ground
Juice from 2 – 3 limes
1 tsp ground chili powder
1 tsp cumin
1¼ tsp. Himalayan salt
½ – 1 whole fresh jalepeno pepper
1 clove garlic
1½ cups water

1. Grind linseeds/flaxseeds.

2. In a food processor, process carrots and bell pepper. Add ground linseed/flaxseed, lime juice, chili powder, cumin and salt. Process until almost smooth.

3. Divide batter in half on two dehydrator trays lined with drying sheets or parchment paper. Spread batter evenly over the entire tray, taking it all the way to the corners.

4. Dehydrate at 47°C/118°F, until firm enough to turn over (3 – 4 hours). Flip onto empty mesh lined trays and peel away drying sheets or parchment carefully.

5. For tortillas, place a round saucer or small plate upside down and score around with a spatula or knife. Use a large plate to make wraps.

6. Gently lift the round tortillas or wraps and place on a fresh (mesh only) tray.

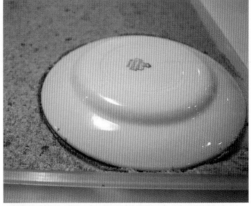

Place a round saucer or plate upside down on partially-dehydrated batter and score around with a spatula or knife.

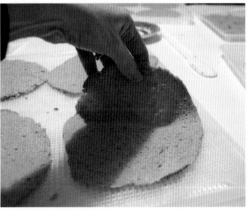

Photos by Geoff Randolph

Gently lift the round tortillas or wraps and place on a fresh mesh tray.

7. Dehydrate tortillas/wraps until they are soft and pliable yet solid and not mushy, approximately 2 – 4 more hours.

8. Using the scraps left over after scoring the circles with the plates (if still moist and pliable), re-spread on a drying sheet placed on top of a new mesh tray. Using a spatula spread the batter evenly as far as it can go (approximately covering 1/3 of the tray). Score this tray into even columns drawing lines horizontally and vertically to make square crackers. Dehydrate this tray for 24 – 36 hours until the crackers are crisp and crunchy.

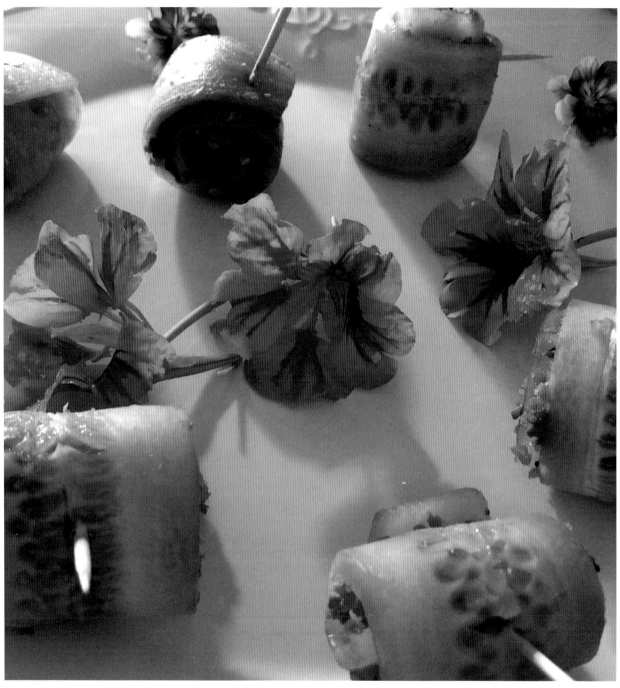

Cucumber Roll Ups with Beet Meat

1 large medjool date, pitted
1 T. chia seeds
3–4 T. water
½ cup almonds, soaked 4–8 hours
½ cup sunflower seeds, soaked 4–8 hours
¼ cup pine nuts, soaked 1 hour
1 beet
2 carrots (or approximately 2 cups carrot
    pulp left over from juicing); divided use
1 small red apple
½ cup left over almond pulp (optional)

1 parsnip
½ cup (total) beet, carrot, apple, parsnip
    juice
2 T. mild white or
    dark miso paste
1 clove garlic, minced
Jalepeno peppers to taste
Himalayan salt
Cucumbers, thinly sliced longways using a
    mandolin

1. Soak nuts and seeds.

2. Juice beet, carrots, apple, and parsnips.

3. Grind nuts in processor, scraping down the sides with a spatula from time to time.

4. Combine the juice pulp with the nut mixture.

5. Put remaining ingredients except for pulp from one carrot (approx. 1 cup) and sliced cucumbers into processor and blend.

6. Slice cucumber longwise on a mandolin.

7. Spoon the beet meat in a line down the center.

8. Sprinkle with carrot pulp.

9. Roll, wrap and pin with toothpick.

Serve with Ginger Yum Yum Sauce (recipe on page 120) and dip the whole wrap generously.

OPTION: Add fresh mint to the sauce.

Not Meat Balls, Beet Balls!

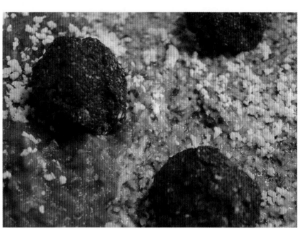

This recipe makes a wonderful meat ball alternative. Serve as a snack with BBQ sauce or use with Raw Marinara Sauce and Walnut Pesto Sauce over raw courgette/zucchini pasta (made using a spriralizer).

Using the recipe for Beet Meat, form into small balls and dehydrate until crisp on the outside (approximately 10 – 12 hours), or to desired dryness.

Looks like ground beef but it's not. It's BEET MEAT!

Photo by Robyn Randolph

Veggie Stir-Unfry

The Ginger Yum Yum Sauce adds a wonderful zip to the fresh crisp flavor of the combined veggies.

        8 green beans, cut on the diagonal into thirds
        6 Chinese peas, cut into thin strips
        1 small red and 1 small orange bell pepper, diced or sliced thin
        ½ head of broccoli including the stems, cut into small pieces
        1 small bunch of baby bok choy, chopped
        Generous handful of mung bean sprouts
        1 carrot, cut on the diagonal into thin circles, grated, or spiral sliced
        Any button mushrooms thinly sliced, or 6 diced shiitakes
        1 tsp. white sesame seeds (optional)
        1 tsp. black sesame seeds (optional)

1. Mix ingredients together in a large serving bowl improvising with any and all of the ingredients depending on what is available.

2. Make a batch of Ginger Yum Yum Sauce (see page 120) and use as much or as little as your taste buds please! Be sure to mix everything together so the sauce coats all the ingredients.

Garnish with lime wedges, snipped chives and sprouts. Serves 1–2.

OPTION: serve over cauliflower or parsnip Nice Rice (see page 145).

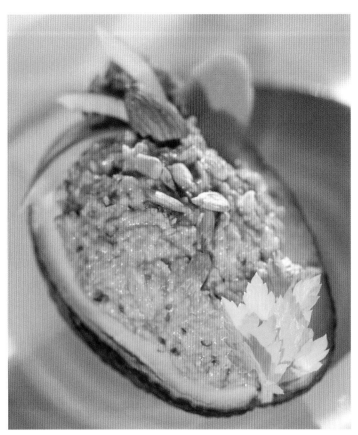

Avocado Boats

½ cup sunflower seeds, soaked
½ cup almonds, soaked
1 large stalk celery
½ of a red bell pepper
1 small tomato
¼ of a red onion
1 clove garlic, minced fine

Make a paté out of the
above ingredients:

1. Soak sunflower seeds and almonds overnight and drain.

2. Dice up small: celery, red bell pepper, tomato and onion.

3. Mix everything together in a food processor and add garlic and Himalayan salt.

Slice 2 ripe avocados in half and stuff with paté! Makes 4 boats.

These are great served with a large salad.

Carrot Walnut Paté

Use this salmon-colored pate to make sushi, to use in wraps or on crackers, with veggies, or as a scoop on top of a fresh garden salad.

1½ cups walnuts, soaked for 6–8 hours
2 T. carrot juice
2 T. nama shoyu or wheat free soy sauce
1 T. lemon juice
½ T. garlic
½ T. ginger
1 cup carrot pulp
⅓ cup sweet yellow onion, minced
¼ cup chopped fresh dill
2 T. fresh-chopped parsley
⅛ tsp. dulse
⅛ tsp. kelp

1. Place drained walnuts, nama shoyu, lemon juice, garlic and ginger into a processor. Blend until smooth.

2. Add remaining ingredients except for carrot pulp and pulse until well blended.

3. Add carrot pulp by hand.

Makes 3½ cups. Lasts in refrigerator for five days.

Kale Chips

Check out our video, *"How To Make Kale Chips,"* on our **Pure Highland Living** channel on YouTube.com: go to YouTube.com in your browser, then search "Pure Highland Living, how to make kale chips" in the YouTube search box.

We think once you try these, you are going to love them. You can never make enough — we recommend you make a triple batch! If you don't already have a dehydrator, Tribest has just set the new standard for state of the art. What a relief to finally have a dehydrator made from BPA-free plastic. This is an important factor in reducing obesogens.

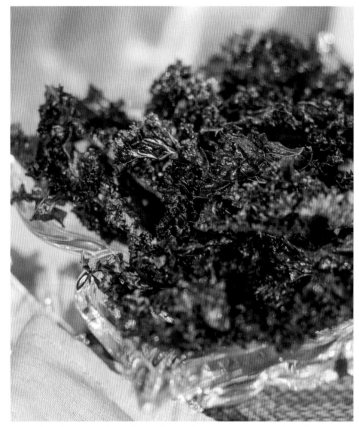

People always ask us how long they can store Kale Chips and still keep them fresh. We haven't a clue, since these disappear right away at our house!

    1 tsp. olive oil
    ¼ cup lemon juice
    1 cup soaked raw cashews or walnuts
    1 red pepper
    2 T. nutritional yeast
    ¼ tsp. cayenne pepper
    ¼ tsp. Himalayan salt

1. Place all ingredients in blender and mix thoroughly.

2. Pour over washed and dried kale and massage well.

3. Place on trays and dehydrate for about 18 hours at 47°C/118°F. Store in glass jar.

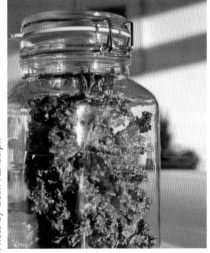

Photo by Geoff Randolph

Mohini's Orange Curly Kale Crisps

Our friend Mohini makes amazing Kale Crisps. They are light, crunchy to perfection after only 4 hours in the dehydrator and very addictive!

Her secret sauce is: fresh orange juice, nutritional yeast flakes, olive oil, salt and pepper, and a little bit of coconut palm sugar. See if you can intuitively sort out the amounts!

NOTE: We love to feature "intuitive chefs" on our blog. If you want to share an intuitive PURE recipe, send us a picture and tell us about you and your recipe! Email us at purehighlandliving@gmail.com.

Butter and Raw Broccoli Bliss (Great for "5 Days")

> 1 head of broccoli broken into bite size dipping pieces
> 4 T. of butter or ghee melted
> Juice of half a lemon
> Several cloves of fresh garlic, minced fine

1. Melt butter.
2. Mix in garlic and lemon.
3. Dip broccoli to your hearts content into the garlic lemon butter. Slurp, slurp, delicious!

Cool Cucumber Butternut Bites

The combination of warm squash on cool cucumber makes this a compelling snack. Just a few bites and you will be hooked!

> ½ butternut squash, baked (this can be done the day before)
> 2 T. butter and/or coconut oil
> Himalayan salt to taste
> Cucumber, sliced into rounds
> Chopped walnuts
> Fresh sage leaves

1. Melt butter and/or oil in fry pan.
2. Scoop out the meat of cooked butternut squash and add to fry pan.
3. Stir to warm and mix with the butter/oil.
4. Add salt and pepper to taste.
5. Spoon on to cucumber rounds.
6. Top with walnuts and garnish with sage.

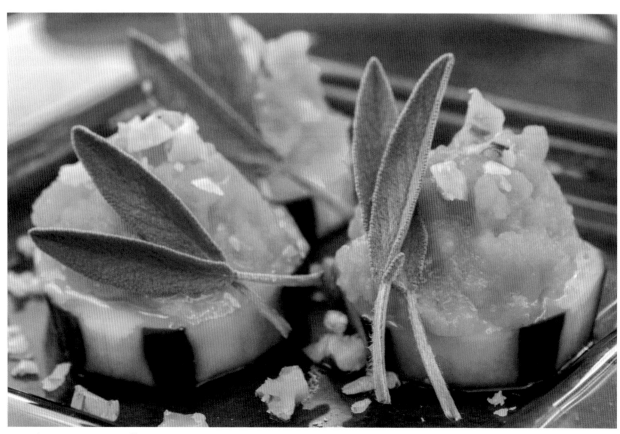

Another intuitive Geoff creation...!

Garlic Grazing Almonds

Warning: These are very addictive. Don't say I didn't warn you! You might want to make a double batch! Trust me on this!

2 ½ cups almonds, soaked 8–12 hours
¼ cup well packed pitted, soft, chopped dates
¼ cup wheat-free tamari
2 T. fresh whey (optional)
2 tsp. fresh garlic, chopped
1 tsp. ginger, finely minced
Pinch of cayenne
Smoked paprika (optional)

1. Strain and rinse the almonds. Set on counter to dry in strainer while you mix the other ingredients together.

2. Place all ingredients except almonds in processor and puree into a paste using the 'S' blade to mix thoroughly.

3. Toss almonds with garlic paste until well coated.

4. Spread almonds onto a dehydrator tray fitted with a drying sheet. We like to use the BPA-free silicon sheets made by Tribest.

5. Dehydrate at 47˚C/118˚F until they are dry enough to remove the underneath sheet. Transfer to a mesh tray and dehydrate another 48 hours or until the almonds are crunchy dry.

Vegan Bliss Burgers

4 T. linseed/flax seed ground in a coffee grinder or in the Personal Blender
½ cup water
1 cup ground sunflower seeds
½ cup walnuts
¼–½ cup sweet onion
1 medium red bell pepper, diced
1 cup carrot pulp from juicing or shredded carrot
2 T. minced parsley
1–2 T. currants
½ cup sundried tomatoes (packed in oil in glass jar; use the tomatoes, not the oil)
Red pepper flakes to taste
Himalayan salt to taste

1. Grind the linseed/flax seed into powder and place into food processor bowl.

2. Add the walnuts and pulse so the walnuts are in very small pieces and mixed with the flax and sunflower.

3. Add all remaining ingredients and blend well. Add small amounts of water if necessary so the blend can be shaped into half-inch thick patties.

4. Dehydrate at 47˚C/118˚F on mesh sheets for 3–4 hours and then turn over. Dehydrate further until firm but not too dry.

5. Serve the patties using a lettuce leaf for the bun. Top with Macadamia Mayonnaise and BBQ Ketchup (see page 122). Garnish with sliced tomato, avocado and sliced onions.

Teriyaki-marinated Mushroom Kabobs with Orange Maple Glaze

This is a brilliant recipe originally inspired by Joshua McHugh of Living Intentions, who I met at the International Festival of Raw and Living Foods about ten years ago. We were both showcasing our recipes, and were both nominated as "Rising Chef Stars" at the festival. Over the years I have made a few adjustments to his recipe, coming up with my own intuitive blend. This recipe goes well with Holiday Nice Rice (recipe follows) and is great for a festive dinner.

Marinade:

1 cup nama shoyu
¾ cup olive oil
1 cup coconut sugar
½ cup pineapple juice
2 T. toasted sesame oil
8 cloves garlic
1 T. fresh ginger, minced (more if you like)
½ T. black pepper
½ fresh jalepeno (more or less,
    depending on how spicy you like it)
    or ½ T. sesame chili oil
1 T. maple syrup

Skewers:

32 cremini mushrooms
1 ripe pineapple cut up in chunks
Basket of cherry tomatoes, cut in half
1 red, orange and yellow bell peppers,
    cut into squares

Glaze:

1 cup orange juice
¼ cup dried pineapple
¼ maple syrup
Pinch of Himalayan salt
½ tsp. lemongrass, zested (optional)
1 tsp. ginger, zested
1 ½ T. white sesame seeds

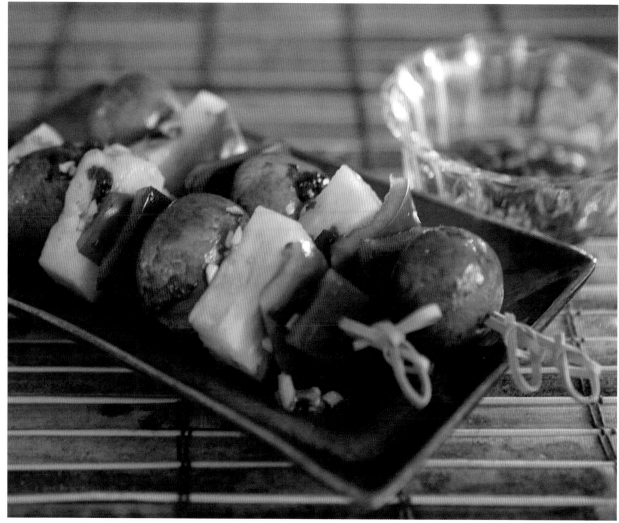

Use a pastry brush to apply the glaze.

Photo by Robyn Randolph

1. Start by soaking dried pineapple in orange juice until very soft (at least an hour).

2. While pineapple soaks, make the marinade by mixing all marinade ingredients in a high-speed blender.

3. In one bowl, cover the mushrooms with enough marinade to coat well. Use the remaining sauce to marinate the sliced tomatoes, peppers and pineapple in another bowl. Marinate for 4 hours at room temperature (stirring from time to time).

4. After marinating, assemble the above onto the skewers and place on a mesh tray lined with a drying sheet. Dehydrate for 2 hours at 47°C/118°F.

5. While the skewers are warming in the dehydrator, prepare the glaze by placing the soaked pineapple and the rest of the glaze ingredients except sesame seeds in a high-speed blender.

6. Strain through a fine mesh sieve. Place the liquid into a large glass pan or pie plate and stir in the sesame seeds.

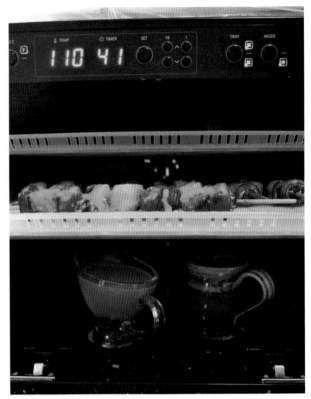

Don't bake, dehydrate!

7. Place on the bottom of the dehydrator and dehydrate 1–2 hours until the liquid turns into a syrup.

When glaze is syrupy, remove skewers and glaze from dehydrator. Brush the glaze on skewers and serve with Holiday Nice Rice.

Holiday Nice Rice

This is a great low-carb alternative to rice and makes a lovely, festive dish served with Marinated Mushroom Kebobs.

> 2 large cauliflower heads,
>   broken into pieces for processing
> 2 parsnips, peeled and cut into chunks
> Handful of fresh mint, chopped
> Himalayan salt to taste
> Pomegranate seeds
> Pine nuts
> Dried, cranberries,
>   sweetened with fruit juice

Garnish with fresh mint leaves and a mound of pomegranite seeds.

1. Using the sharp "S" blade, process the cauliflower with the mint until it resembles fluffy rice. Place into a mixing bowl.

2. Process the parsnips the same way and add to bowl.

3. Stir in the salt, pomegranate seeds, pine nuts, and cranberries in any amounts you like (use your intuitive cooking skills for this)!

OPTION: Use the left over marinade from making the Marinated Mushroom Kebobs over the rice.

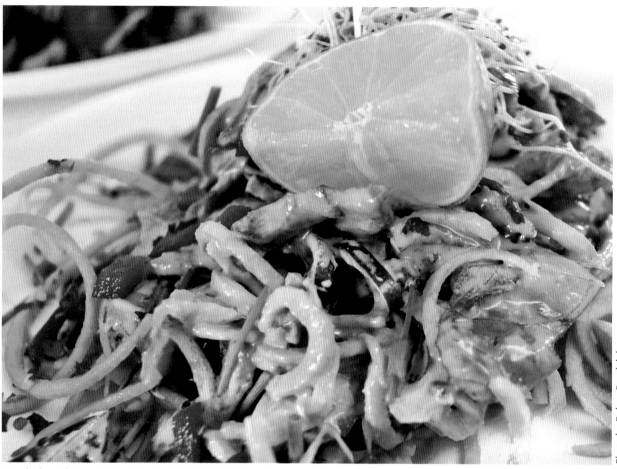

Made by Claire of Meadowlark Café in Edinburgh.

PURE Pad Thai with a Lime Twist

Even though this recipe requires a bit of prep time, it is so worth it! The marinade is so delicious you will want to drink it up. You can use it for salad dressing too.

Pad Thai

- 1 green courgette/zucchini, julienned or turned into "angel hair" with a spiral slicer
- 1 yellow courgette/zucchini, prepared the same way
- 2 large carrots, julienned
- 1 red, 1 orange and 1 yellow bell pepper, sliced into thick strips
- 1 large green apple, julienned (with skin on)
- 1 cup purple cabbage, sliced paper-thin
- Small bunch of fresh cilantro/coriander
- 1 cup bean sprouts
- ½ cup black sesame seeds

Chili Lime Sauce

- ½ cup raw almond butter
- 1½ tsp. grated ginger, skin and all
- 3 T. lime juice
- ¼ cup coconut water (more if needed)
- 2 cloves garlic
- 2 T. Namu shoyu
- 1 T. maple syrup
- 1 Thai dragon chile pepper, Serrano pepper or pepper of your choice
- 5–10 fresh mint leaves
- 1 T. olive oil

1. Mix all ingredients for Chili Lime Sauce in a blender.
2. Prep vegetables according to ingredients list and place in a large bowl.
3. Toss with Chili Lime Sauce.
4. Garnish with black sesame seeds and lime wedges.

OPTION: For a beautiful presentation, carefully remove leaves of a purple cabbage and arrange around a platter, mounding the Pad Thai on top of the leaves.

146

Green Thai Vegetable Curry

By intuitive raw chef Julie Howes.

Chop vegetables of preference or the following:

Rocket (aragula)
Tomatoes
Cucumber
Broccoli
Watercress
Spinach
Celery
Pineapple

NOTE: Adjust amounts to suit how many people you are serving.

For Green Thai Curry Sauce enough to serve two, put in blender:

One ripe avocado
1 T. coconut oil (approx)
1 T. apple cider vinegar
1 garlic clove
3 T. cold pressed olive oil
½ tsp. Himalayan salt (or to taste)
1 tsp. spoon turmeric powder
2 medjool dates soaked until soft in half cup of filtered water

NOTE: Try it without chili or extra garlic first, and add chili and/or more garlic if you would like it hotter/spicier.

Blend until creamy. Put salad and vegetables in a pretty bowl, pour the sauce on top and serve.

OPTION: Garnish with fresh lime slices.

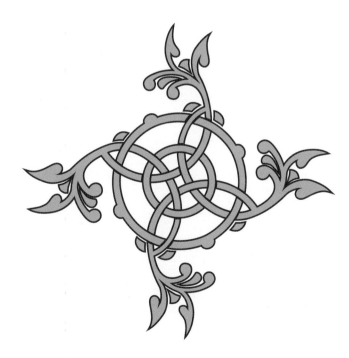

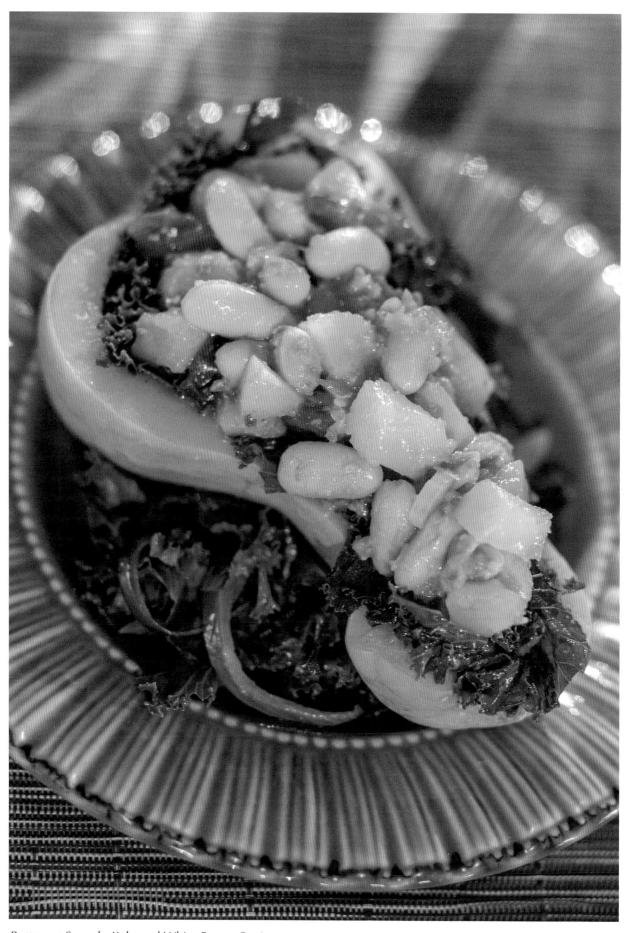

Butternut Squash, Kale and White Beans. Recipe on page 155.

Lemony Garlic Braised Greens

Organic butter
1 diced red onion
1 T. finely chopped clove of garlic
Juice of two lemons
Any combo of kale, collards, and chard, cut up into ribbon strips
Sesame seeds

1. Sauté onion in butter and add water if you wish for more moisture.

2. Next, add garlic and lemon juice, sautéing until garlic and onions have cooked well, adding water and more lemon juice as needed.

3. Wash but don't drain the greens and add to skillet.

4. Place a lid on the skillet and turn heat down to low. Cook until tender.

5. Sprinkle with sesame seeds.

Serves 2–4.

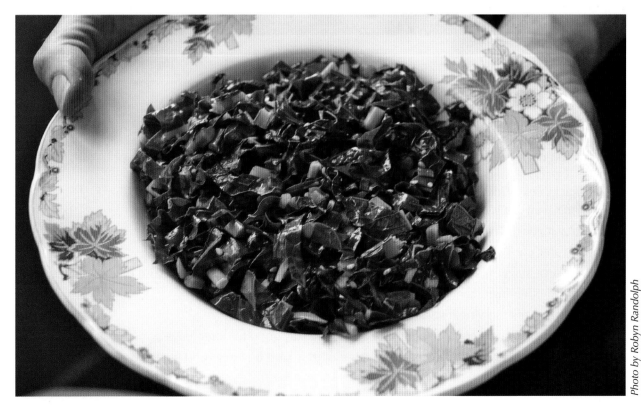

Use kitchen scissors to snip the kale into ribbon strips.

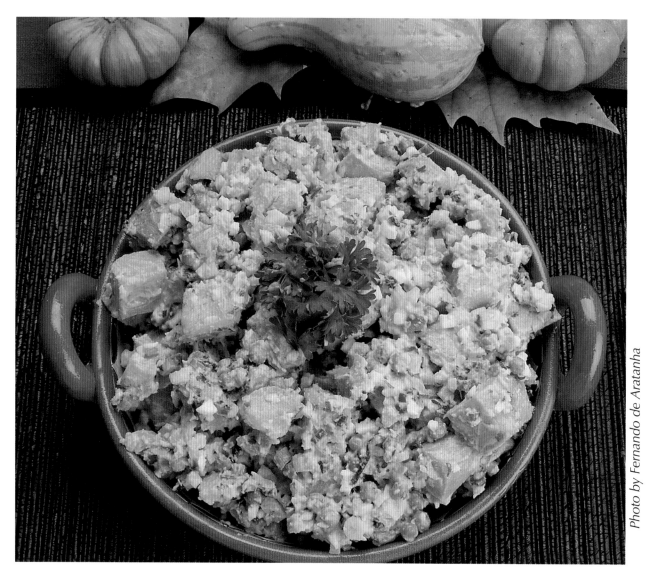

Yum Yum Yam Salad

6 large garnet yams (or sweet potatoes)

¾ cup Macadamia Mayonnaise (see page 122), or mayonnaise of your choice (in the USA, Vegenaise is a good option)

1 bunch green spring onions, sliced

Small bunch of parsley, diced fine

½–1 package of organic frozen peas

5 sticks celery, diced into small pieces

Himalayan salt to taste

1. Cut yams into chunks and steam them with skins on until soft but still firm.

2. Let yams cool and then peel off skins.

3. In a large stainless steel bowl, cut yams into chunks and mix with mayonnaise of your choice.

4. Add all other ingredients and stir gently.

5. Place in a nice serving dish and garnish with parsley sprigs.

6. Store in an air-tight container in fridge and it will stay good for three days.

NOTE: For non-vegans, you can slice up three or four hard boil eggs and gently toss in.

Serves 6–8.

Oat Groat Veggie Risotto with Yum Yum Sauce

We believe eating grains should be restricted due to the inflammation that can tend to happen with eating grains. However, we have found oat groats as an occasional replacement for brown rice to be a satisfying and health benefitting option. Oat groats are unprocessed whole oats.

    1 cup oat groats, soaked overnight and rinsed well
    2 cups water
    1 strip of kombu seaweed
    2–4 cloves garlic

1. Place oat groats in water and bring to a boil. Snip kombu into little pieces with kitchen scissors and add as it begins to cook. Also throw in garlic cloves.

2. Simmer on low for about 30 minutes or until cooked.

3. Use enough Home Base Sauce (recipe page 119) to sauté the following:
    6 shiitake mushrooms, sliced
    3 medium tomatoes, chopped (or sundried tomatoes)
    1 red and 1 yellow onion, diced
    1 bunch broccoli
    2 small zucchinis, sliced

1. 4. After all veggies are cooked crisp-tender, turn off heat and add desired amount of Ginger Yum Yum Sauce (see page 120). Blend with cooked oat groats. Serves 2–4.

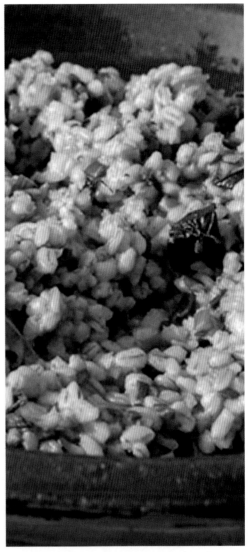

Oat Groat Risotto is great served with a garden-fresh salad.

Quinoa Delight

We believe eating grains should be restricted, due to the inflammation that grains can cause. Technically, quinoa is a seed and a good source of plant protein.

    1 onion, diced
    5 or 6 shiitake mushrooms, cut into small pieces
    Generous handful of string beans, cut into thirds (eliminate the tips first)
    2 large stalks of broccoli, chopped
    Slivered almonds
    1 cup quinoa, soaked for 4–8 hours
    Home Base Sauce (see page 119)

1. Soak quinoa four to eight hours. Drain and rinse.

2. Heat quinoa in 2 cups water just to boiling, then simmer over low heat until all water is absorbed. Be sure to check on it regularly, as it cooks in about 20–30 minutes.

3. Shake up Home Base Sauce and pour enough to coat a pan generously.

4. Sauté onions and mushrooms. Once onions are soft, add green beans and broccoli.

5. Cover and cook on low until crisp and tender.

6. Turn off heat, add cooked quinoa to pan, and toss well.

Serve with slivered almonds. Serves 2–4.

NOTES: For non-vegans, adding a small amount of organic feta cheese at Step 6 makes for a yummy, creamier taste. Be sure to toss well.

Currants or raisins are also a wonderful addition, and makes this more kid-friendly too!

Baked Neep Slices (Swedes/Rutabagas)

I could eat these every night. Geoff made them up when we found that neeps are in abundance here in the Highlands! In the spirit of local and sustainable eating, we especially encourage our Scottish friends to try this! I suggest you double the amount, because no doubt you will want more!

Start with:

½ of a large neep, thinly sliced, about 1/8 inch thick or less

Coating:

1 T. butter
1 T. coconut oil
1 T. hot water
1 tsp. garlic powder
⅛ tsp. Himalayan salt

1. Blend coating in personal blender.

2. Dip sliced neep pieces into it to coat the pieces.

3. Spread on cookie sheet and bake at 400F (200C) for 15–20 minutes.

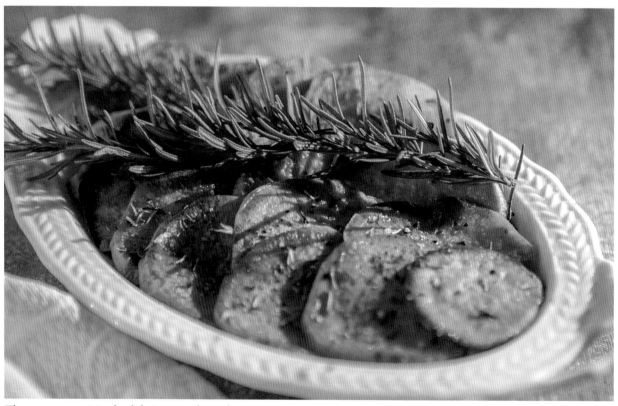

These are surprisingly delicious and satisfying.

Spicy Turmeric Groats

2 cups oat groats (could also use brown rice)
1 T. coconut oil
2 tsp. turmeric
½ tsp. red pepper flakes
2 T. shredded dry coconut
8 dates, pitted and finely chopped
¼ tsp. Himalayan salt
Lime wedges

1. Rinse the oat groats or rice.

2. Drain and add 3 cups of water. Bring to a boil then cover and simmer for 35–40 minutes.

3. After groats or rice is cooked, add the other ingredients and stir well to evenly distribute everything.

4. Garnish with lemon wedges.

NOTE: Eat grains sparingly.

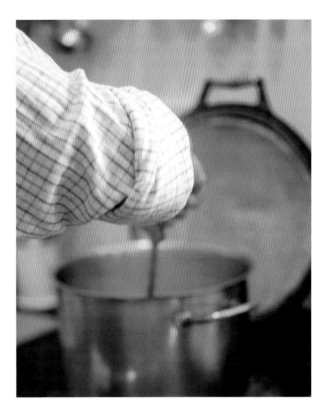

Get Smashed – Garlic Cauliflower

When I serve this with gravy on top, many people do not even realize that it is cauliflower and not mashed potatoes!

2 heads cauliflower
¼ cup organic olive oil
1 small clove garlic or ½ tsp. garlic powder
Himalayan salt to taste
Any herbs or spices you like on mashed potatoes
Organic butter or ghee
Small amount of plain rice milk, goat milk, or water

1. Steam cauliflower until soft and tender.

2. Place all ingredients in processor and add small amounts of rice milk or water until cauliflower resembles mashed potatoes.

A real crowd pleaser! Serves 4.

Root Vegetable Roast in a Green Olive Glaze

Comfort food at its healthiest and best. Root vegetables roasted on a cold winter's eve sends waves of delight to the heart of your belly. I love throwing in the apples and olives to add a sweet and pungent part to the equation. This is great served with a big salad.

2 parsnips
1 rutabaga, diced (also known as a swede)
3 garnet yams, peeled and diced
2 beets, diced
2 Fuji apples, diced
12–20 cloves of garlic
⅓ cup water
1 cup gourmet green olives of your choice
⅓ cup olive oil
1 tsp. Italian seasoning

1. Place first seven ingredients into a casserole pot and toss with olives, oil, water, and seasoning.

2. Cover with a lid and bake in the oven at 190°C/375°F until everything is soft in the middle when poked with a fork. Serves 2–4.

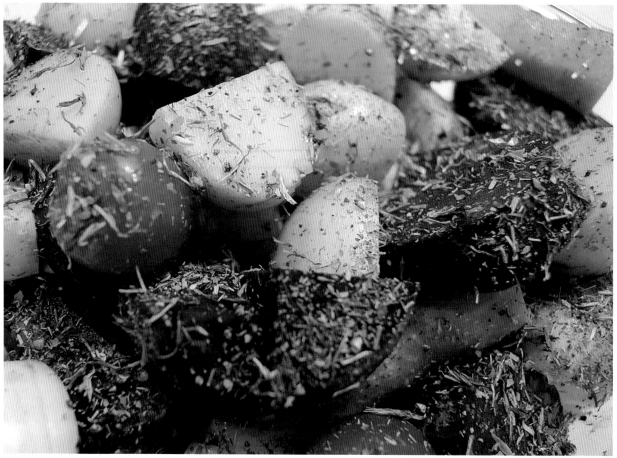

Root Vegetable Roast with wildflower herbs and spices.

Butternut Squash, Kale & White Beans

I enjoy this recipe so much when I want greens and beans! The combination is just perfect for a satisfying warm meal on a cold night. See picture of this recipe on page 148.

2 cups dried white beans
2 carrots, sliced
3 stalks celery, sliced
Himalayan salt and garlic powder to taste
1 large butternut squash
1 small red onion, diced
1 bunch of kale, cut into small pieces
2 T. Home Base Sauce (see page 119)
1 can of salt-free diced stewing tomatoes
1 T. olive oil

1. Measure out 2 cups beans and place in pot.
2. Add 6 cups of water and throw in carrots, celery, garlic powder and salt to taste. Cook until beans are tender.
3. While beans cook, steam the squash until tender.
4. Next, sauté red onions in Home Base Sauce. After onions are soft, add kale and cover with a lid. Turn heat down and sauté until kale is tender.
5. In a skillet, heat olive oil and add stewing tomatoes.
6. Remove outer skin of butternut squash and cut into small chunks.
7. Add to the tomatoes. Cook only long enough to mix the two together to warm all the way through.
8. Using a slotted spoon, remove three or four spoonfuls of cooked beans, including as many pieces of carrots and celery as possible. Blend in a processor or blender with a small amount of cooking water.
9. Drain the remaining beans, carrots and celery and discard the cooking water.
10. Add blended beans back into whole beans. Season to taste.
11. On a plate or in a bowl, begin with a portion of kale to form the bottom layer. Next add a layer of the tomato and squash mixture, and finally a topping of beans.

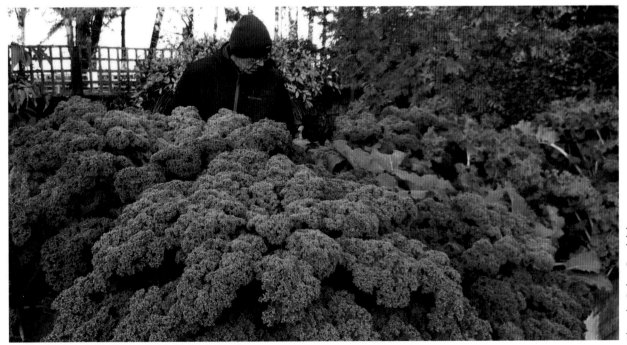

Geoff and his massive crop of winter kale.

Photo by Robyn Randolph

Mashed Yellow Peas with Roasted Peppers

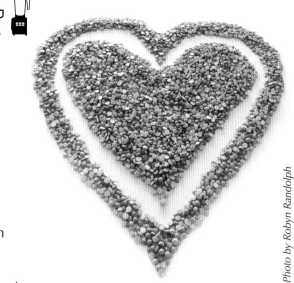

Yellow split peas are a great PURE food addition, providing several health benefits These include maintaining proper blood sugar balance, which is essential for health as well as weight loss.

    2 cups yellow split peas
    6 cloves garlic
    Red and orange bell peppers
    Juice of 1 lemon
    Butter
    Himalayan salt and pepper to taste

1. Place split peas in pot with garlic cloves and pour in enough water to have at least two inches covering the peas. Cook until very very soft.

2. While peas are cooking, cut peppers into quarters and place in a baking dish. Squeeze lemon juice over the peppers and dot with butter. Bake at 190°C/375°F until browned.

3. Drain excess water from peas and blend peas in blender/processor.

4. Take skins off baked peppers and cut into small pieces. Blend peppers into mashed peas.

We "heart" yellow split peas!

Photo by Robyn Randolph

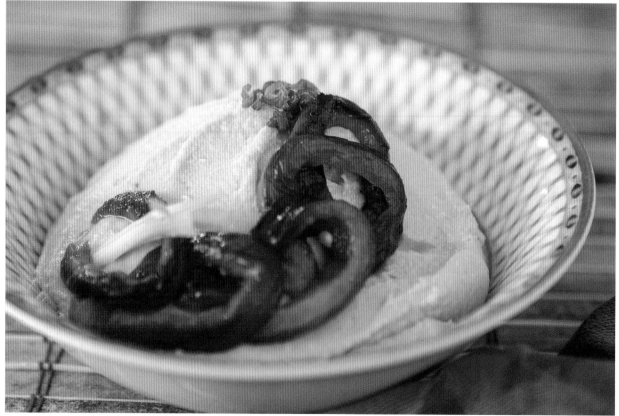

Save some of the chopped roasted peppers as a garnish and sprinkle with snipped chives.

Photo by Robyn Randolph

Gluten-free Courgette Walnut Pear Bread

The pears make this gluten-free bread extra yummy. If you have never cooked with coconut flour before, you might be pleasantly surprised to find such a great gluten-free option.

        1 medium to large courgette (zucchini)
        ¾ cup coconut flour
        1 tsp. baking soda
        ½ tsp. Himalayan salt
        1 T. cinnamon
        ½ tsp. nutmeg
        3 T. coconut sugar or maple syrup
        5 large organic eggs
        2 T. coconut oil or organic butter
        1 large pear, diced
        ½ cup walnuts, chopped
        3 T. of water if necessary
        Extra cinnamon for the top

1. Preheat oven to 175°C/350°F and grease a square pyrex baking dish or bread pan.

2. Shred courgette.

3. Mix together all dry ingredients in one bowl (except for pears and walnuts).

4. Mix eggs well and add maple syrup (if you aren't using coconut sugar). Melt butter or coconut oil and add, mixing all together well.

5. Mix liquids in with the dry ingredients.

6. Fold in the diced pear and chopped walnuts, mixing well.

7. Pour into greased pan and sprinkle some extra cinnamon across the top.

8. Bake 40–50 minutes.

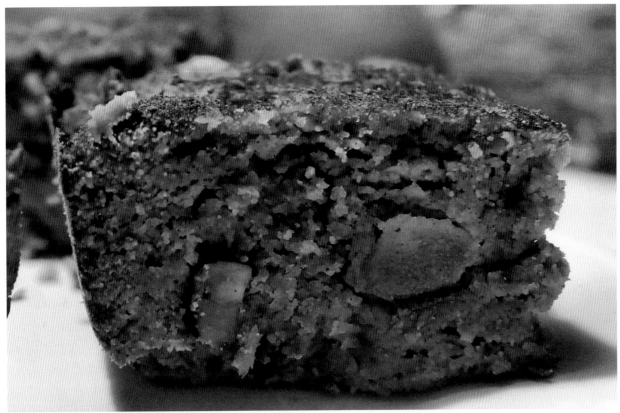

Photo by Robyn Randolph

The warm baked pears really make this so irresistable when it comes fresh from the oven—and with a dab of organic butter, even better!

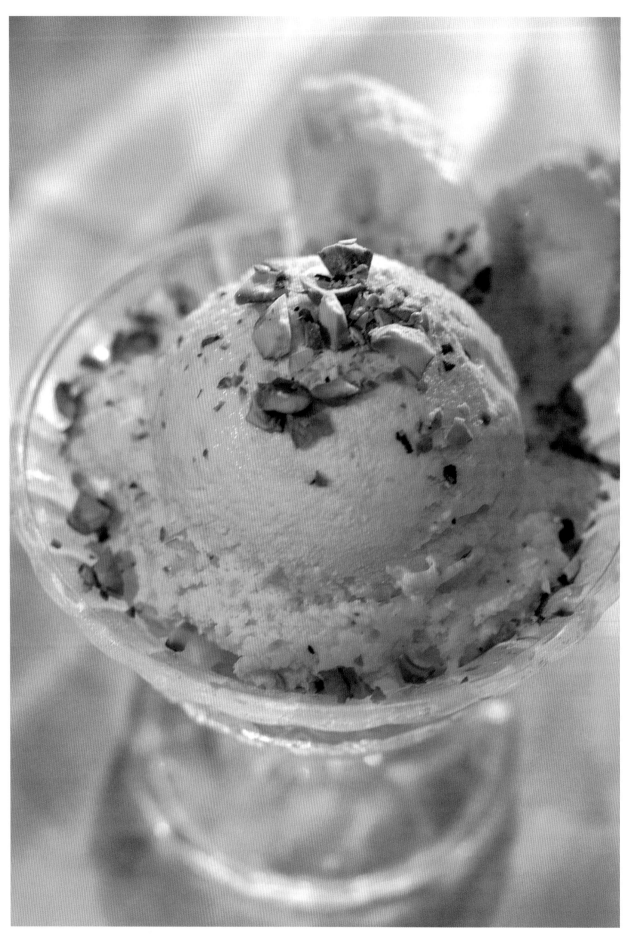

Banana Cardomom Ice Cream. Recipe on page 162.

A Few PURE Raw Sweet Treats

For best results, restrict sweets to once per week maximum
during the 21 Days of Transformation, and only eat sweets on a "5 day."

Classic PURE Raw Chocolate by Rosie Balyuzi

If you LOVE chocolate…

For balance, high anti-oxidants and the sheer pleasure of healthy chocolate, be sure to add this into your 21 Days of Transformation!

    70g raw virgin coconut oil
    70g organic cocoa butter
    45g raw organic cocoa powder
    45g organic lacuma powder (it's a popular South American fruit)
    2 T. raw runny honey (or an alternative sweetener of choice, such as rice or date syrup, stevia, coconut sugar)

Necessary Implements:
    Wooden spoon
    Glass bowl
    Saucepan
    Chocolate bar moulds, or Tupperware sandwich box bases; these make excellent moulds

1. Place the glass bowl over a saucepan of water on the hob (stove). Bring the water to the boil and as soon as it boils, take off heat.

2. Put coconut oil and cocoa butter into the glass bowl, still over the pan, and stir gently with a wooden spoon until it is melted to a clear liquid.

3. Stir in the honey in same way until dissolved.

4. Sieve in the cocoa powder and lacuma powder in stages, stirring in gently until it forms melted chocolate.

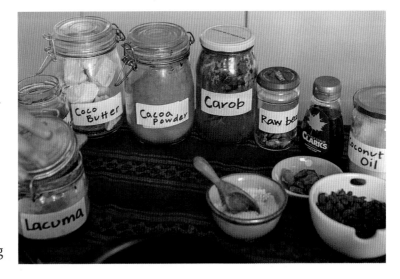

5. Before pouring into tupperware bases or moulds, any special extras can now be added to the mix, such as dried fruits, nuts, seeds, spirulina powder, and/or edible-grade essential oils (no more than 8 drops per batch). It is up to your imagination as a chocolatier!

NOTE: This is a great way to add spirulina! Just stir it in and make sure it gets blended well.

6. Now pour chocolate into moulds, to the thickness of an average bar and refrigerate for one hour. Wrap and keep refrigerated in between eating.

This chocolate lasts up to four weeks in the fridge.

Raw Banana Walnut Fudge Brownies

Brownies

¾ cups walnuts
½ cup or ground almonds or pecans, or leftover pulp from making almond milk
1¼ cups dates
⅓ cup cocoa
1 tsp vanilla
2 T. maple flavored agave
Pinch Himalayan salt

OPTION: add 1 tsp. carob mint spirulina or plain spirulina (see Chapter 6, *Get Equipped*).

1. Mix all together and put in pyrex dish.

2. Slice bananas and place in rows on top.

3. Make frosting and coat evenly over bananas.

Frosting

4 T. coconut butter
2 T. raw honey
4 tsp cocoa powder
Pinch Himalayan salt
1 tsp water more if needed

4. Top with ½ T. chopped walnuts.

5. Put in fridge to set for about 2 hours.

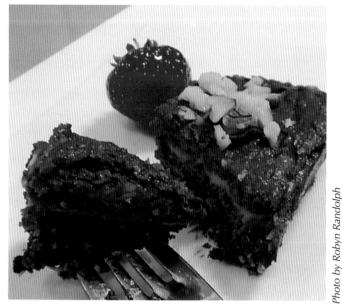

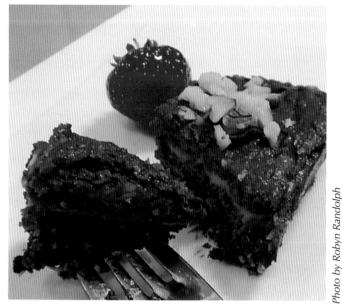

Adding spirulina to these brownies is a great way to mask the taste of the algae while adding superior nutritional benefits.

Photo by Robyn Randolph

Spirulina Goji Berry Balls

10 dates, pitted
Tahini
Carob mint spirulina or plain spirulina (see *Get Equipped*)
Goji berries and or currants
Pecans, chopped small

1. Begin by processing dates.

2. Add 1 T. tahini (more if you like).

3. Add 1–2 tsp. spirulina and blend in food processor.

4. Pulse in as many goji berries and or currants as you would like.

5. Place chopped pecans on a plate and roll the balls in the pecans to coat.

OPTION: Add organic cocoa powder.

Carob Almond Squares

2½ T. carob powder
6 T. coconut oil
4 T. agave, maple or date syrup (your choice)
½ tsp. Himalayan salt
1 cup almonds, soaked 6–8 hours, rinsed,and drained

1. In a food processor, finely grind ¾ cup of the soaked/drained almonds. Chop the other ¼ cup into small bits and set aside.

2. Mix everything else together in a processor.

3. Press into a small square glass dish.

3. Top with the chopped almonds.

4. Place in freezer to set up for at least an hour, then cut into squares and serve.

OPTION: replace the almonds with walnuts.

Chocolate Spirulina Freezer Fudge

6 T. coconut oil
1 T. cocoa powder
1 T. carob mint spirulina or plain spirulina (see *Get Equipped*)
¾ cup chopped brazil nuts
½ cup currants or dried raspberries (optional)
4 T. agave, maple or date syrup
Pinch of Himalayan salt

1. Mix all ingredients together in a processor.

2. Press into a small square glass dish.

3. Place in freezer for at least an hour, then cut into squares and serve.

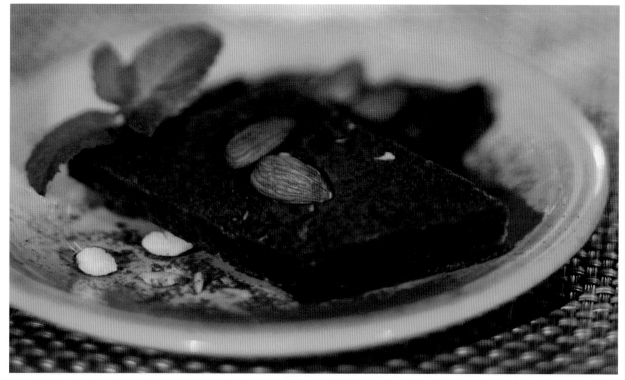

Carob Almond Squares are another great way to slip in the benefits of spirulina while masking the algae taste.

Coconut Applesauce

Perfect for kids of all ages! Great gourmet baby food for the wee ones. Also a nice way to use those abundant autumn apples.

> 2 apples
> 1 tsp. cinnamon
> ½ tsp. vanilla
> 3 room temperature, soft dates (pitted)
> Fresh coconut water

Mix all ingredients together in a processor, adding small amounts of coconut water as needed.

Serves 2.

Clever Carob Pudding

This is for those who don't do chocolate. Who would have thought that avocado would be the star of this unusual pudding? Trust me, the kids won't know! You have to make this to taste how positively pleasant this pudding is. This wows the guests too!

> 2 T. carob powder
> 1 cup water or coconut water
> 1 tsp. vanilla
> ¼ tsp. cinnamon
> 10 soaked and pitted dates
> 1 avocado
> 4 sliced strawberries

1. In a food processor, combine all ingredients except for the strawberries, dates and avocado.

2. While processor is running, slowly add dates and avocado until smooth.

3. Alternate layers of strawberries with pudding in long-stemmed glasses and top with berries.

Serves 2.

NOTE: Adding more coconut water will turn this from pudding into a sauce you can pour over Banana Cardamom Ice Cream.

Banana Cardamom Ice Cream

See the picture of this amazing treat on page 158!

> 5 ripe bananas, broken into 4 or 5 pieces and frozen
> 3 pods of cardamom (remove the seeds and discard the pods)
> ¼ – ½ cup coconut water or almond milk
> 2 tsp. coconut oil
> Pistachio nuts, chopped (optional)

1. In a high speed blender, mix ¼ cup coconut water or almond milk with the cardamom seeds and coconut oil until seeds are broken down well.

2. Add pieces of frozen banana and blend to desired consistency, adding more liquid if necessary.

3. Sprinkle with chopped pistachio nuts.

Serves 4.

OPTION: Add 1 T. carob mint spirulina or plain spirulina (see Chapter 6, *Get Equipped*).

Meyer Lemon-Lavender Cheesecake 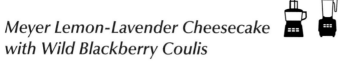 *with Wild Blackberry Coulis*

This divine non-dairy recipe was originally created by my friend, Joshua McHugh of Living Intentions. It is the perfect sweet treat for those who love cheesecake or don't fancy chocolate. You will be amazed how incredible it tastes!

1 cup pecans
1 cup shredded coconut
½ cup pitted dates
¼ tsp. Himalayan salt
1¾ cup cashews ground up into a fine powder (in blender and then set aside in a bowl)
1¼ cup young coconut meat or 200g packaged pure creamed coconut
⅔ cup Meyer lemon juice
6 T. honey
6 T. coconut oil
2½ T. chopped ginger
2½ T. vanilla extract
1¼ tsp. dried lavender flowers
2 T. lemon zest (5–6 lemons)
10 oz wild blackberries (can use frozen if need be)
3 T. agave nectar
Wild berries and fresh lavender for garnish

For crust:

1. Place pecans, dates and salt into processor and blend into a fine consistency.

2. Press pecan mixture into a spring form pan.

For lemon cream:

3. In a high-speed blender, place coconut meat, lemon juice, honey, coconut oil, ginger and vanilla and blend until smooth.

4. Add cashews and lavender and blend until smooth.

5. Add lemon zest and blend on low speed. Using a spatula remove mixture from the blender and smooth on top of the crust.

6. Place cake into the freezer for 2 hours. Thaw for 15 minutes before serving.

For blackberry coulis:

7. Place blackberries and agave nectar into a high speed blender and blend until smooth. Strain coulis through a fine sieve or nut milk bag. Pour into a squeeze bottle.

To assemble:

8. Place slice of cheesecake in the center of a plate. Squeeze coulis onto the cake and plate creating an artistic pattern. Garnish with fresh berries and lavender.

Ginger/Vanilla Cheesecake with Raspberry-Chocolate Swirls and Chocolate Pecan Crust

I invented this cheesecake to make for Christmas dinner at Newbold House where we were guest chefs on Christmas Day 2013.

NOTE: I like to use a fluted metal pie pan with a removable bottom. It makes things so much easier when it comes time to cut and serve—trust me on this! It is worth the investment. You will use this over and over for years to come!

    1¾ cup pecans
    ¾ cup shredded coconut
    3 T. cacao powder
    1 ½ tsp. Himalayan salt (divided use)
    6–8 soft dates
    1 T. maple syrup (for crust); 1/3 cup raw honey or maple syrup (for filling)
    2 T. + 1 tsp. vanilla (divided use)
    2 cups cashews, soaked with enough water to cover for at least one hour and then drained
    1¼ cup young coconut meat or package of PURE creamed coconut (condensed coconut found in
       200g packages, for those in the UK who can't access fresh coconuts)
    3 T. coconut oil
    3 T. really warm water (to help melt the coconut oil)
    2 T. chopped fresh ginger

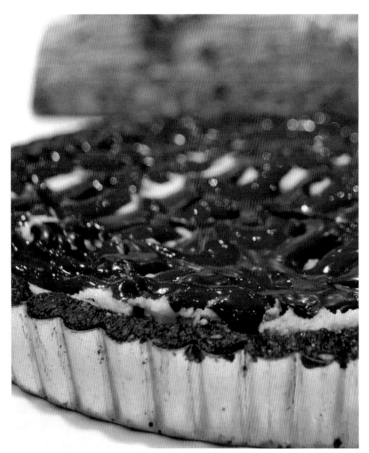

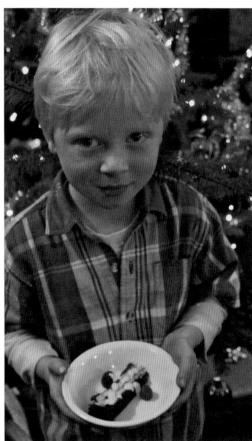

Photos by Robyn Randolph

LEFT: *Geoff thinks this is my best dessert creation... let me know what you think.*
RIGHT: *This was a big hit with young and old at Newbold House Christmas dinner.*

Crust:

1. Oil pan with enough melted coconut oil to cover the bottom and sides.
2. Process the pecans fine but not enough to become a paste or butter. Blend in shredded coconut, 3 T. caco powder, salt, dates, 1 T. maple syrup, and 1 tsp. vanilla. Process until fully combined.
3. Press into pie pan using the back of a spoon. Build up sides of crust to top edge of pan.
4. Place in freezer while making filling and toppings.

Ginger/Vanilla Cheesecake Filling:

5. if using young coconut meat, process until smooth.
6. Add the soaked and drained cashews, two T. vanilla, the coconut oil, ⅓ cup honey or maple syrup, the salt, warm water ,and ginger and process all together.

    While processing, stop and scrape down the sides to help mix all ingredients really smooth. Be sure to take a sample taste. It is so delicious you will want to eat it just like this, but don't give in to temptation—proceed!
7. Measure out a heaping cup of the cheesecake mixture and set aside. Spread the remaining cheesecake batter into pan, using a spatula to make it smooth and flat.
9. Place back in freezer while you make the chocolate and raspberry sauces.

The Sauces:

Raw Cacao Sauce

> ¾ cup raw cacao powder
> ¼ cup + 1 T. maple syrup
> 2 T. melted coconut oil
> 6 T. water

Mix well in a high speed blender.

Raw Raspberry Sauce

> ½ package thawed, frozen organic raspberries. *NOTE:* Be sure to drain off excess juice after thawing, to make it as thick as possible.
> 2 T. agave or maple syrup

Mix in a high speed blender.

The Fun Part!

1. Pour the chocolate and raspberry sauces into separate squirt bottles.
2. Using half of each kind of sauce, make alternating parallel lines with raspberry and cacao sauces across the top of the pie. Don't worry about how neat or straight they are.
3. Using a chopstick, drag the tip in lines across your swirl patterns.
4. Place back in freezer for half an hour, then fill pan with the reserved

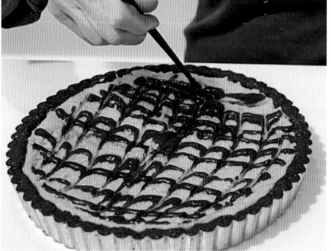

Photo by Geoff Randolph

cheesecake batter and then repeat steps 2 and 3 with the rest of the two sauces on the top.

Freeze until you are ready to serve. Garnish with mint and fresh raspberries. For a festive Christmas dessert, garnish with berries and holly sprigs in the center.

Rawbannutty Pie

This recipe was inspired by a delicious Bannoffee Pie we ate at the Mustard Seed in Inverness, Scotland. I wanted to come up with a dairy-free, PURE version of the recipe, and I could not be more pleased with this. I used the basic ingredients from the Meyer Lemon-Lavender Cheesecake adding, of course, lots of ripe bananas!

1 cup pecans
½ cup pitted dates
¼ tsp. Himalayan salt
1¾ cup cashews, ground to a fine powder in blender and set aside
1¼ cup young coconut meat, or 200g package of pure creamed coconut
3 T. maple syrup
3 T. coconut oil
4 ripe bananas for filling, plus 1–2 sliced bananas,
    depending how much you want (see Step 6 below)
1 T. chopped ginger
Pinch Himalayan salt
2½ T. vanilla extract
Sliced bananas
Dusting of cocoa powder

Crust:

1. Place pecans, dates and salt into processor and blend into a fine consistency.

2. Press pecan mixture into a springform pan.

Banana cream:

3. In a high-speed blender, place creamed coconut or young coconut meat, bananas, maple syrup, coconut oil, ginger, pinch of salt and vanilla and blend until smooth.

4. Add ground cashews and blend until smooth.

5. Using a spatula remove two-thirds of the mixture from the blender and smooth on top of the crust.

6. Place a solid layer of banana slices on top.

7. Cover the bananas with the remaining one third of the cream.

8. Place cake into the freezer for 2 hours. Thaw for 15 minutes before serving.

9. Lightly dust the top of the cake with raw cocoa powder, and garnish with fresh flowers and lavender.

Mac-a-roons

3 cups shredded coconut
1½ cups almond flour or left over pulp from almond milk
1 cup maple syrup
⅓ cup coconut oil
1 T. vanilla
½ cup ground macadamia nuts
½ tsp. vanilla powder
½ tsp. Himalayan salt

1. Mix all together in a food processor.

2. Form into balls. Place on mesh sheets and dehydrate at 47°C/118°F for 8–24 hours, depending on how firm and crunchy you like them.

Spir-a-roons

3 cups shredded coconut
1¼ cups raw organic cocoa powder
4 T. spirulina
1 cup maple syrup
⅓ cup coconut oil
1 T. vanilla
½ cup ground macadamia nuts
½ tsp. Himalayan salt

1. Mix all together in a food processor.

2. Form into balls. Place on mesh sheets and dehydrate at 47°C/118°F for 8–24 hours, depending on how firm and crunchy you like them.

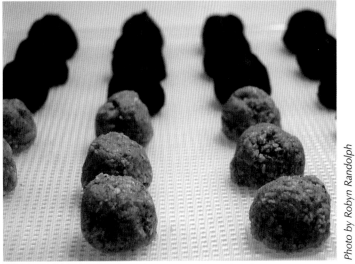

Photo by Robyn Randolph

Mac-a-roons in front and spir-a-roons in back, ready to dehydrate!

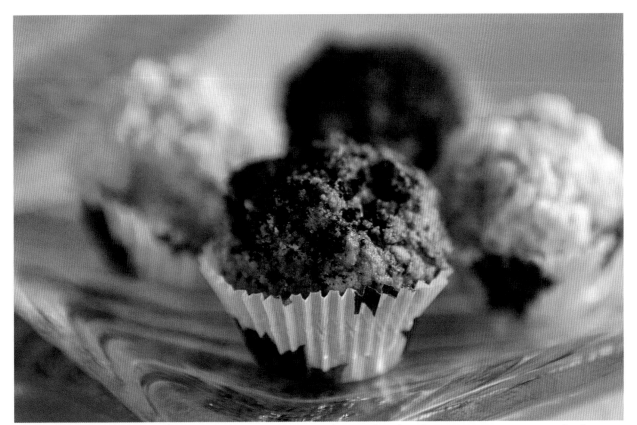

The cocoa and coconut hide the strong taste of the spirulina and makes this sweet treat power-packed with antioxidants.

Chocolate Mousse

> 3 medium-sized ripe avocados
> ¾ cup cacao (or substitute carob)
> ½ cup maple or date syrup, can also use ½–1 cup coconut sugar
> 1 tsp vanilla powder or ½ tsp liquid vanilla
> ½ tsp cinnamon
> Pinch of Himalayan salt
> ¾ cup water

In a food processor, puree all ingredients until smooth, slowly adding the water last until you get your desired consistency.

Garnish with fresh raspberries, cacao nibs or mint. 3 1– cup servings.

Banana Fingers

Slice bananas on the diagonal and put a dollop of the mousse above on each slice. !

Chocolate Mousse Pie

Crust

> 1¾ cup dry macadamia nuts
> ¼ cup pitted dates
> 1 cup almond pulp
> ⅛ tsp. Himalayan salt
> Pinch of cayenne pepper

1. Process mac nuts, then add dates, almond pulp and salt into processor and blend into a fine consistency.

2. Press mixture into a springform pan.

3. Fill with **Chocolate Mousse** (above).

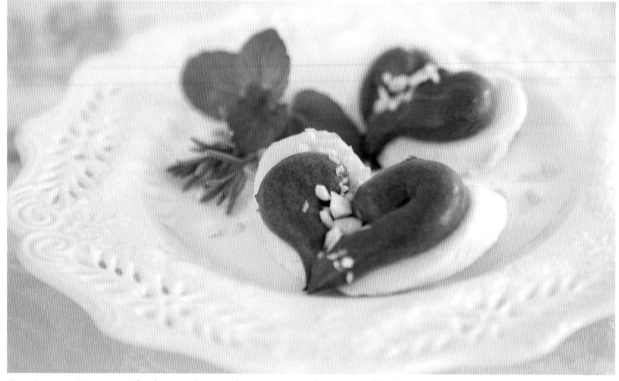

Top Banana Fingers with chopped macadamia nute and a piece of fresh mint. Yum!

Cashew Whipped Cream

Use this (or the coconut version below) in place of dairy whipped cream. Perfect for vegans!

Cashews, soaked
Maple syrup to taste
1 tsp. vanilla
A pinch of Himalayan salt

Soak cashews in coconut water enough to cover for at least an hour, then drain. Process everything together, and enjoy!

Coconut Whipped Cream

Fresh coconut meat
Shredded coconut
Soaked dates (optional)
Vanilla
Agave
Pinch of Himalayan salt

Process all ingredients together. Thicken by adding shredded coconut to your desired consistency.

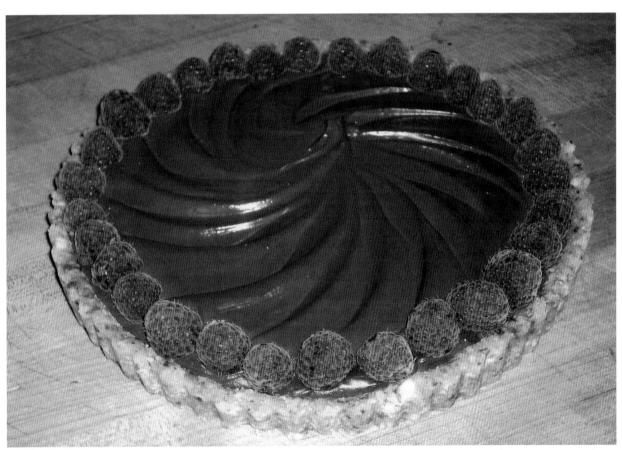

Everyone is always surprised to find out the mousse is made with avocados!

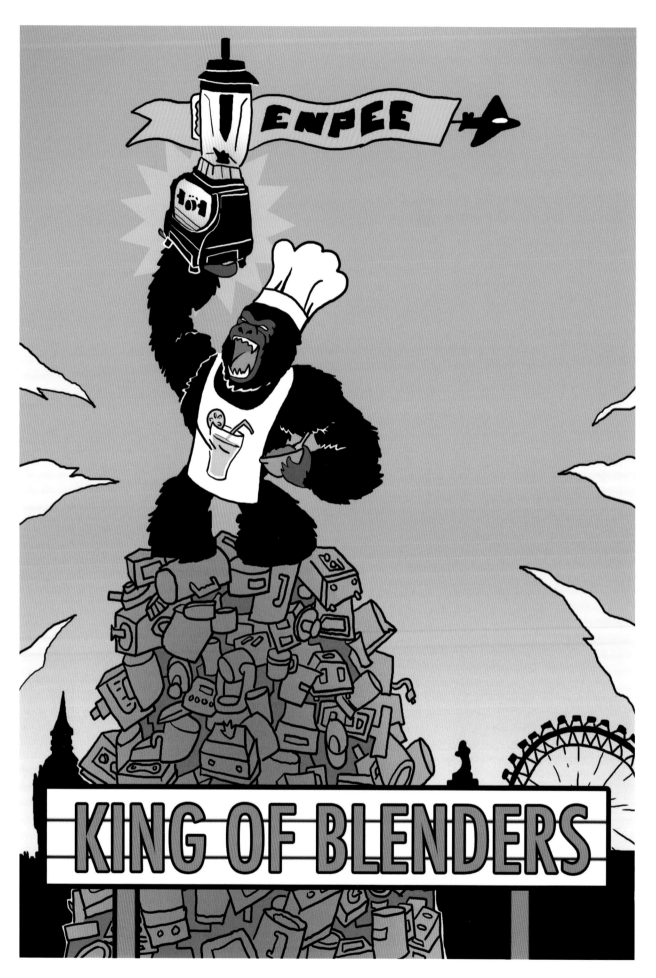

Chapter 6 - Get Equipped

We are passionate about sharing what we love with others who want to make this a lifestyle and need assistance getting set up. We appreciate the opportunity to work with you personally. We are here to help you create the healthy lifestyle that best suits you.

On our websites, you will find the latest, state-of-the-art equipment and organic, PURE, whole foods and super food supplements, including healthy oils. When you order through us, you get our personal help and guidance as well as having real, live people to follow up on your orders! We price competitively with Amazon and accept PayPal as well as online banking options. We will not be undersold, so feel free to do a price match with us.

You can see our complete store on our website: **purehighlandliving.com**. We sell all Tribest kitchen equipment, both in the UK and the USA.

We appreciate your business and referrals, as this is how we fund publishing our books and talks. Thank you for being a part of our PURE Food Revival Revolution! Let us know if we can help.

To order spirulina and barley grass powder:

    USA: **phporder.com/ProductPage.aspx?ItemID=37&ID=rawsome**

    UK: **purehighlandliving.com/shop/superfoods** or
               platinumuk.biz/ProductPage.aspx?ItemID=461&ID=rawsome

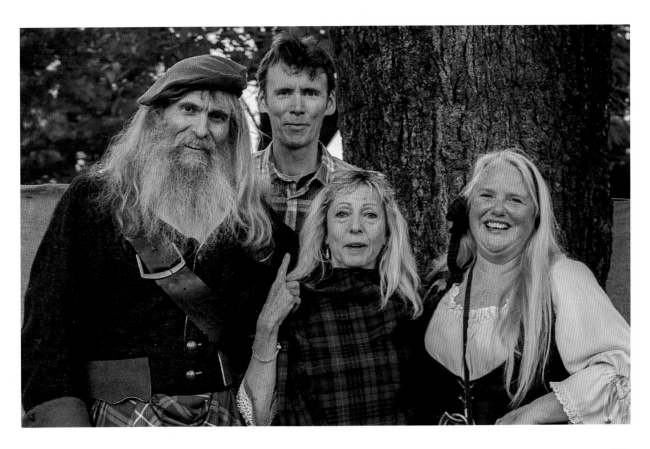

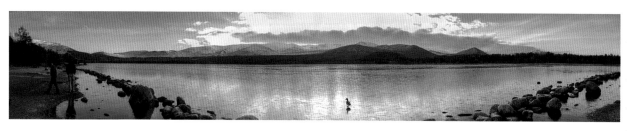

ꝒURE Resources We Appreciate

In the UK:

Connage Highland Dairy

For those using dairy products we believe it is essential to buy only organic (as chemicals bond to fats).

"This is a traditional family-owned, fully organic business, situated on our family farm, Milton of Connage at Ardersier. All our products are fully traceable and we apply excellent quality controls from 'cow to cheese'. We can assure the highest standard of animal welfare and care for our cows, continuing the attention to detail into our cheeses."

connage.co.uk

Creelers

Creelers of Skye is world famous for their simple French cooking using top quality, local, pure Scottish ingredients. We use their Cajun spice mix for our raw flax crackers. A must if you love seafood and are on the West Coast of Scotland.
skye-seafood-restaurant.co.uk

Earth Ways

Ludwig specializes in helping you to design and create your own vibrant, thriving, highly-productive natural ecosystem and edible landscape. Any size of project is suitable, from urban terraces and
rooftops to large farms and estates. Permaculture design, forest gardening, ethical tree care, invasive species control and organic growing principles are all used to transform conventional landscapes into rich, self-regulating habitats – natural havens that nurture and sustain people and wildlife alike.

earth-ways.co.uk

Ellishadder Art Café

Situated on the spectacular North East cost of Skye, Ellishadder Café uses local and seasonal organic produce served in a relaxed atmosphere featuring quality art work.

ellishadderartcafe.co.uk

The Fresh Network

World's most comprehensive raw and living foods organization, and publishers of Get Fresh!
fresh-network.com

Graham's Organic Scottish Butter

"The Graham Family has been dairy farming for five generations, so it really is in our blood. Our butter is made from our own fresh organic cream, lightly churned to produce a butter that is fabulously rich and creamy. Good taste is in our nature."

grahamsfamilydairy.com/our-ranges/butter/scottish-organic/

Herbal Heritage Scotland

Claire MacKay (BSc), Medical Herbalist and founder of Herbal Heritage Scotland, notes:
"It has become a matter close to my heart to maintain research and to collate much of the existing resources and available research including a wealth of Gaelic, orally collected accounts that is the very roots of a tradition, traceable in our Scottish heritage as far back as 5000 years ago.
Our native plants have preserved humankind down the centuries, and it is my intention, not only to use the skills I have gained to heal people naturally, within our communities, but also to preserve the carefully cultivated plant knowledge of our Scottish heritage. Shop online for her organic, healing teas."

herbalheritage.co.uk

Hiddenglen Organic Holidays

Located on Laikenbuie Organic Farm in Nairn (Scottish Highlands), a little peace of heaven where you can experience the wildlife and farm animals on a tranquil organic croft, and yet be close to many attractions and exciting places to visit in the Highlands of Northern Scotland. Locally, look for Laikenbuie free-range eggs and lamb.

hiddenglen.co.uk
youtube.com/watch?v=USQd4dSKXyA

Knockfarrel Organic Farm/Produce

Jo Hunt runs this family run croft, nestled beneath the Iron Age hill fort of Knockfarrel, producing salads, herbs, vegetables, eggs, and preserves, and raising pigs.

knockfarrel.com

Living Food Festival

Held annually at Cawdor Castle, this is the Highland's original food and drink festival with an emphasis on artisan, organic, and local produce enhancing the profile of the area. It provides a memorable day out for the family and new markets for local producers, while showcasing sustainable credentials.

cawdorcastle.com/livingfood/about.cfm

Mcleod Organics

The Highlands' original box delivery scheme. A family farm that has been delivering since October 1998, with a proud history.

"We remain fully committed to bringing the freshest, most local possible, and absolutely 100% organic products to your doorstep for the best value we can manage."

macleodorganics.co.uk

Natural Vegetable Company

An organic farm located on the southern edge of Inverness farmed by Maggie Sutherland. She is a Soil Association registered organic producer committed to natural horticultural production. She offers a complete range of seasonal produce from the field to the consumer. Visit the web site to see box schemes that can be ordered online.

natvegco.com

Newbold House

A community located in Forres, Scotland, that is a retreat, workshop centre, and B&B with 7 acres of walled organic gardens in Forres in Northern Scotland, close to Findhorn in Morayshire. See web site for list of upcoming events. This is one of our favorite places to hold workshops.

newboldhouse.org

Poyntzfield Herb Nursery

Specialising in the cultivation of herb plants and seeds using organic and biodynamic principles. They offer for sale over 400 varieties, either from the nursery or by mail order (including overseas countries). The herbs originate from countries all over the world, but they include in their range plants native to Scotland that have herbal properties. The nursery is situated on the Black Isle – a low peninsula surrounded by sea lochs, hills and mountains. Because of the high latitude and long winters, all plants are hardy, suitable for almost any garden.

"We have been growing herbs organically since 1976 and the quality of many species has been enhanced by propagating only from plants known to have hardiness, health, vigour, resistance to pests and diseases, good scent, colour and flavour."

poyntzfieldherbs.co.uk

Riverdale Centre

Complete wellbeing in one place in the heart of Inverness. Complementary therapies, health foods, organic café and juice bar.

therapies-inverness.co.uk

Strathconnon Highland Organix

Fabulous jams, jellies, chutneys and original and unusually fabulous organic preserves made by Jacqui McKinnon from ingredient grown on her organic farm.

facebook.com/strathconon.highlandorganix

TIO Ltd *(This Is Organics)*

One of the leading organic food producers and suppliers in the UK, located in Forres, Scotland.

"We are organic root vegetable specialists and we can also source other organic food products via our established network of growers and producers. One of our biggest strengths is the fact that we own our own farms and processing factory. This ensures that we can control the quality of our products, from seed to shipping."

tio.co.uk

Velocity Café and Bicycle Workshop

A social enterprise in the heart of Inverness, aiming to increase access to the joys that being on a bicycle, eating delicious healthy food and telling stories can bring. The café plays an integral role and their methods of delivery are uncompromising; wholesome, healthy, local food, at accessible prices, in an inclusive and welcoming space. They use local organic produce grown by Maggie Sutherland of Natural Vegetable Company.

velocitylove.co.uk/cafe/

Organic Food Stores in the Highlands and Morayshire

We so appreciate each one of these businesses for supplying PURE, healthy food in an area where sometimes finding organic can be a bit of a challenge!

The Health Shoppe
20 Baron Taylor's St.,
Town Centre, Inverness IV1 1QG
Phone: 01463 233104

Highland Whole Foods Unit 6
13 Harbour Road, Inverness IV1 1SY
Phone: 01463 712696

The Phoenix, The Park, Forres,
Highlands and Islands IV36 3TZ
Phone: 01309 690110

Skye Delights, 9 Leopold St.
Town Centre, Nairn IV12 4BE
Phone: 01667 452874

In the USA:

Anderson Almonds: Organic almonds by the case (25 lbs.) nice price reduction! **andersonalmonds.com 209-667-7494**

Bariani Olive Oil: Unheated, unfiltered, stone-pressed organic olive oil. **barianioliveoil.com 916-689-9059**

Bauman College: Hollistic Nutrition and Culinary Arts Certification Programs. **baumancollege.com**

Bella Vita Lifestyle Education Center: Residential 10-day cleanse, detox and rejuvenate program with a biblical diet base. **modernmanna.org/categories/ BellaVita-%252d-Lifestyle-Center/**

Big Tree Organics: Organic almonds at great prices. **bigtreeorganic.com 209-669-3678**

The Date People: Offering a huge selection of fresh organic dates. **datepeople.net 760-359-3211**

The Hippocrates Health Institute: Offering residential programs lasting anywhere from one to three weeks, sometimes even longer. This allows you to learn, absorb, and implement a new set of lifestyle strategies at a deep and lasting level. Four powerful nutritional approaches taught there are: shifting from burning carbs to burning fat for fuel; eating raw foods (especially sprouts); avoiding sugar; including fruit; lowering the overall animal protein content in your diet. **hippocratesinst.org 888-228-1755**

Optimum Health Institute: Reasonably priced retreat, healing and nutritional health resort teaching and providing raw living foods lifestyle. **optimumhealth.org 800-993-4325**

New Natives: Highest quality seeds and supplies for sprouting. **newnatives.com**

Purium Health Products: Exceptional green products (kamut, spirulina, barley grass) as well as other high quality "super food" supplements. **phporder.com/rawsome**

Sun Organic Farm – Full online organic shopping great for all dry goods. **sunorganicfarm.com**

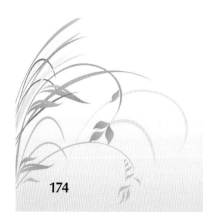

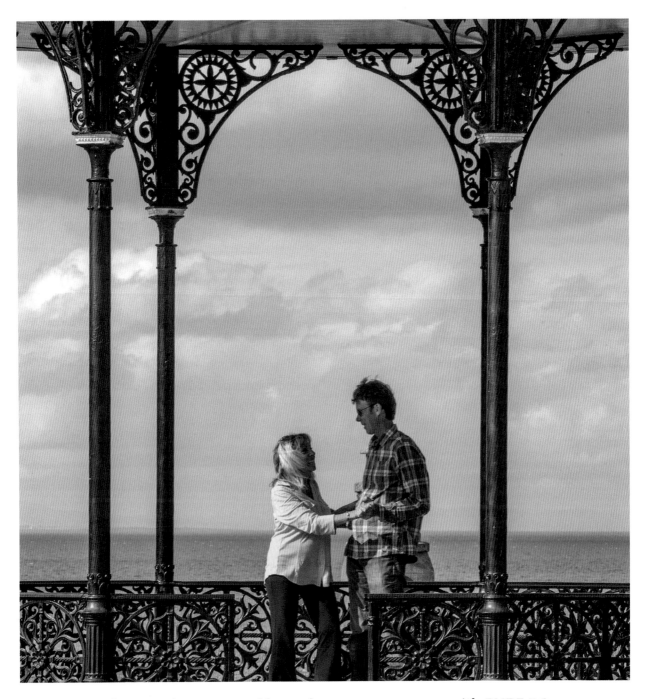

Please write to us and let us know your success with PURE 5:2

purehighlandliving@gmail.com

Eat well and be well! Cheers,

Robyn and Geoff Randolph

If you would be interested in attending a **PURE 5:2 Healthy Holiday Retreat** with us in the Highlands of Scotland please contact us. We do private and group retreats and we are also available for speaking and teaching engagements.

If you like this book, we would love to know about it! Please give us a review on Amazon!

Join us in our PURE food revival by sharing this with a friend you think could benefit! If each one can teach one, we can make a difference in the health of the world!

References:

Chapter 1: Why PURE?

1. Excitotoxin: "A substance added to foods and beverages that literally stimulates neurons to death, causing brain damage of varying degrees. Can be found in such ingredients as monosodium glutamate, aspartame (NutraSweet), cystein, hydrolyzed protein, and aspartic acid." From the back cover of *Excitotoxins: The Taste That Kills* by Russell Blaylock, MD.

2. *Americans Eat Their Weight in Genetically Engineered Food;* article by Renée Sharp, Director of Research, Environmental Working Group, October 15, 2012.

3. *Impacts of genetically engineered crops on pesticide use in the U.S.—the first sixteen years;* article by C. M. Benbook, Environmental Sciences Europe 2012.

4. *Genetic Roulette: The Documented Health Risks of Genetically Engineered Foods;* Jeffrey M. Smith, Gene Ethics Limited, 2007.

5. *GM Soy Linked to Illnesses in Farm Pigs;* article by Dr. Eva Sirinathsinghji, Institute for Science in Society, June 27, 2012.

6. *Long-term toxicity of a Roundup herbicide and a Roundup-tolerant genetically modified maize;* article by Gilles-Eric Seralini et al., Food and Chemical Toxicology, Vol. 50, Issue 11, Nov. 2012.

7. *Answers to Critics: Why there is a long term toxicity due to a Roundup-tolerant genetically modified maize and to a Roundup herbicide;* Seralini, G.-E. et al. Food and Chemical Toxicology, 2012.

8. *The Island Where People Forget to Die;* article by Dan Buettner, The New York Times, October 24, 2012.

9. *Phosphate Additives in Food—a Health Risk,* article by E. Ritz, K. Hahn, M .Ketteler, M. Kuhlmann, and J. Mann, aerzteblatt.de/int/archive/article/119592, 2012.

10. *Review of Harmful Gastrointestinal Effects of Carrageenan in Animal Experiments;* article by J. K. Tobacman, Environmental Health Perspectives, October 2001.

Chapter 2: How, What and Where to Get Pure Foods

11. *Vegetarian Myths;* article by Stephen Byrnes, ND, PhD, RNCP, 2000. **mercola.com,**

12. *It's the Beef: Myths & Truths about Beef;* article by Sally Fallon and Mary G. Enig, PhD, 2000. **westonaprice.org/food-features/its-the-beef**

13. **phytochemicals.info** Website devited to information on phytochemicals

14. *Eating less butter and more fat;* chart from Butter through the Ages web site: **webexhibits.org**.

15. *Omega-6 Fats in Processed and Deep Fried Foods Can Massively Increase Your Heart Disease Risk;* **articles.mercola.com/sites/articles/archive/2013/02/21/omega-6-dangers.aspx#_edn1**

16. *Why Butter is Better;* article by Sally Fallon and Mary G. Enig, PhD, January 2000, **westonaprice.org/food-features/why-butter-is-better**

17. *The Incredible Health Benefits to You of Traditionally Fermented Foods;* **articles.mercola.com/sites/articles/archive/2004/01/03/fermented-foods-part-two.aspx**

18. *When Never Ever To Use Fish Oil;* **articles.mercola.com/sites/articles/archive/2010/10/16/rudi-moerck-on-fish-oil.aspx**

19. *Metabolic effects of krill oil are essentially similar to those of fish oil but at lower dose of EPA and DHA, in healthy volunteers;* Ulven, Kirkhus, Lamglait, Basu, Elind, Haider, Berge, Vik, and Pedersen, 2010. **ncbi.nlm.nih.gov/pubmed/21042875**

Recommended Reading on Enzymes:

20. *Food Enzymes—The Missing Link to Radiant Health;* by Humbart Santillo, Lotus Press, 1993.

21. *The Complete Book of Enzyme Therapy;* by Dr. Anthony Cichoke, Avery Trade, 1998.

22. *The Effect of Dietary Composition on the Pancreatic Enzymes;* article by Grossman, et al, The American Journal of Physiology, 1943.

23. *Enzyme Nutrition—The Food Enzyme Concept,* by Dr. Edward Howell, Avery Publishing Group 1995.

24. *On the Synergistic Effects of Enzymes in Food with Enzymes in the Human Body. A Literature Survey and Analytical Report;* L. J. Prochaska, W. V. Piekutowski, 1994. **ncbi.nim.nih.gov**

Chapter 3: How and Why to Do PURE 5:2

25. *Changing perceptions of hunger on a high nutrient density diet;* Article by Joel Fuhrman, Barbara Sarter, Dale Glaser, and Steve Acocella. 2010. **nutritionj.com/content/9/1/51**

26. *Does hunger and satiety drive eating anymore? Increased eating occasions and decreasing time between eating occasions in the United States;* article by Barry M. Popkin and Kiyah J. Duffey, American Journal of Clinical Nutrition, 2010.

27. *Dietary energy density in the treatment of obesity: a year-long trial comparing 2 weight-loss diets;* article by Julia A. Ello-Martin, Liane S. Roe, Jenny H. Ledikwe, Amanda M. Beach, and Barbara J. Rolls, American Journal of Clinical Nutrition, 2007.

28. *Achieving Great Health,* Bob McCauley, Spartan Enterprises, 2005.

29. *Comparison with ancestral diets suggest dense acellular carbohydrates promote an inflammatory microbiota, and may be the primary dietary cause of leptin resistance and obesity;* article by Ian Spreadbury, 2012. **ncbi.nlm.nih.gov/pmc/articles/PMC3402009/**

30. *Agrarian diet and diseases of affluence – do evolutionary novel lectins cause leptin resistance?* Tommy Jönsson et al, BMC Endocrine Disorders, 2005. **biomedcentral.com/1472-6823/5/10,**

31. *Effects of a high-protein ketogenic diet on hunger, appetite, and weight loss in obese men feeding ad libitum;* article by Alexandra M. Johnstone et al, American Journal of Clinical Nutrition, 2011.

32. *Carbohydrate restriction has a more favorable impact on the metabolic syndrome than a low fat diet;* J. S. Voltek et al, 2009. **ncbi.nlm.nih.gov/pubmed/19082851**

33. *Carbohydrate Restriction, as a First-Line Dietary Intervention, Effectively Reduces Biomarkers of Metabolic Syndrome in Emirati Adults;* M. Fernandez et al, The Journal of Nutrition, 2009

34. *Limited Effect of Dietary Saturated Fat on Plasma Saturated Fat in the Context of a Low Carbohydrate Diet,* C. E. Forsythe et al, 2010. **ncbi.nlm.nih.gov/pubmed/20820932**

35. *Eating, exercise, and "thrifty" genotypes: connecting the dots toward an evolutionary understanding of modern chronic diseases;* M. V. Chakravarthy, F. W, Booth; 2004. **ncbi.nlm.nih.gov/pubmed/14660491**

36. Introduction to *Evolutionary Medicine and Health;* by W. R. Trevathan, E. O. Smith, and J. J. McKenna. Oxford University Press, 1999, pp. 3-6.

37. *Autophagy in the Pathogenesis of Disease,* article by B. Levine and G. Kroemer, *Cell* (periodical), 2008.

38. *Short-term modified alternate-day fasting: a novel dietary strategy for weight loss and cardioprotection in obese adults;* K. Varady, et al, American Journal of Clinical Nutrition, 2009.

39. *Intermittent versus daily calorie restriction: which diet regimen is more effective for weight loss?* K. Varady, Obesity Reviews. 2011.

40. *Intermittent fasting dissociates beneficial effects of dietary restriction on glucose metabolism and neuronal resistance to injury from calorie intake;* article by R.M. Anson et al, National Academy of Sciences (US), 2003.

41. Caloric restriction and intermittent fasting: Two potential diets for successful brain aging; B. Martin et al. Ageing Research Reviews, August 2006.

42. *Modified alternate-day fasting regimens reduce cell proliferation rates to a similar extent as daily calorie restriction in mice;* K. Varady, The FASEB Journal, June 2008.

43. *Effect of intermittent fasting and refeeding on insulin action in healthy men;* N. Halberg et al, Journal of Applied Physiology, December, 2005.

44. *Obesogens: An Environmental Link to Obesity;* Wendee Holtcamp, Environmental Health Perspectives, February 2012.

45. *Canaries in the coal mine: a cross-species analysis of the plurality of obesity epidemics;* Yann C. Klimentidis et al, Proceedings of the Royal Society of Biological Sciences, November 2010.

46. *Prenatal concentrations of PCBs, DDE, DDT and overweight in children: a prospective birth cohort study;* D. Valvi et al. Environmental Health Perspectives, October 2011.

47. *Chronic Exposure to the Herbicide Atrazine Causes Mitochondrial Dysfunction and Insulin Resistance;* S. Lim et al. April 2009. **plosone.org/article/info:doi/10.1371/journal.pone.0005186**

48. *Prenatal Exposure to Perfluorooctanoate and Risk of Overweight at 20 Years of Age: A Prospective Cohort Study,* T. Halldorsson et al, Environmental Health Perspectives, May 2012.

49. *Concentrations of Urinary Phthalate Metabolites Are Associated with Increased Waist Circumference and Insulin Resistance in Adult U.S. Males;* R. Stahlhut, et al, Environmental Health Perspectives, March 2007.

50. *The gut microbiota as an environmental factor that regulates fat storage,* F. Backhed et al. Proceedings of the National Academy of Sciences, November 2004.

51. *Weight gain in the first week of life and overweight in adulthood: a cohort study of European American subjects fed infant formula;* N. Stettler, V. A. Stallings, A. B. Troxel, J. Zhao, R. Schinnar, S. E. Nelson, et al, April 2005. **circ.ahajournals.org/content/111/15/1897.full**

52. *Consumption of monosodium glutamate in relation to incidence of overweight in Chinese adults: China Health and Nutrition Survey (CHNS);* K. He et al, American Journal of Clinical Nutrition, June 2011.

53. **truthinlabeling.org** —names of ingredients that contain processed free glutamic acid (MSG).

Cross Reference Articles:

54. *Health at Every Size: The Surprising Truth About Your Weight;* Linda Bacon, BenBella Books, 2010.

55. *The Obesity Myth: Why America's Obsession with Weight is Hazardous to Your Health;* Paul Campos, Gotham Books2004.

56. *The epidemiology of overweight and obesity: Public health crisis or moral panic?* Paul Campos, Abigail Saguy, Paul Ernsberger, Eric Oliver, Glenn Gaesser, International Journal of Epidemiology, December 2005.

57. *The Fat Chick Works Out! Fitness that's Fun and Feasible for Folks of all Ages, Shapes, Sizes and Abilities;* DePatie, Jeanette, Real Big Publishing, 2011.

58. *Health implications of obesity: An alternative view;* P. Ernsberger, P. Haskew, Journal of Obesity and Weight Regulation, 1987.

59. *Fatness, Fitness & Health: A Closer Look At The Evidence;* A. Glenn, Absolute Advantage 5, 2006.

60. *Confronting the failure of behavioral and dietary treatments for obesity;* David M. Garner, Susan C. Wooley, Clinical Psychology Review 11, 1994.

61. *Health At Every Size,* J. Robison, Absolute Advantage 5, 2006.

62. *Weighing Both Sides: Morality, Mortality, and Framing Contests over Obesity;* A. C. Saguy, Journal of Health Politics, Policy and Law 30, 2005.

63. *Just the Weigh You Are: How to Be Fit and Healthy, Whatever Your Size;* Steven Jonas, Linda Konner, Rux Martin/Houghton Mifflin Harcourt 1998.

Additional Books and References:

Achieving Great Health by Bob McCauley

Big Fat Lies by David Gillespie

Don't drink A1 Milk by Brent Bateman

Ignore the Awkward, How the Cholesterol Myths Are Kept Alive by Uffe Ravnskov

In Defense of Food by Michael Pollan

Ischaemic heart disease, Type 1 diabetes, and cow milk A1 beta-casein; M. Laugesen and R. Elliott, The New Zealand Medical Journal Jan. 2003.

Nourishing Traditions by Sally Fallon and Mary Enig

Omega Six, The Devil's Fat by Robert Brown

RawSome Recipes by Robyn (Boyd) Randolph

Reader's Digest's *Foods That Harm, Foods That Heal*

Sweet Fire by Mary Toscano

The Coconut Oil Miracle by Bruce Fife

The Devil in the Milk by Keith Woodford

The Great Cholesterol Con by Malcolm Kendrick

The Green Food Bible by David Sandoval

The Oiling of America by Sally Fallon

The Paleo Answer by Loren Cordain PhD

The Paleo Solution – The Original Human Diet by Robb Wold

The Palm Oil Miracle by Bruce Fife

The Warrior Diet by Ori Hofmekler

We Want Real Food by Graham Harvey

Wild Fermentation by Sandor Ellix Katz and Sally Fallon

Website Sources

fooducate.com

blog.fooducate.com/about-2/product-grading/

seedsofdeception.com

naturalnews.com
store.naturalnews.com/Superfoods_c_4.html
naturalnews.com/039993_fooducate_GMO_smart_phone.html#ixzz2R2mjJ7ox

mercola.com

westonaprice.org

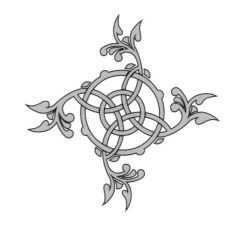

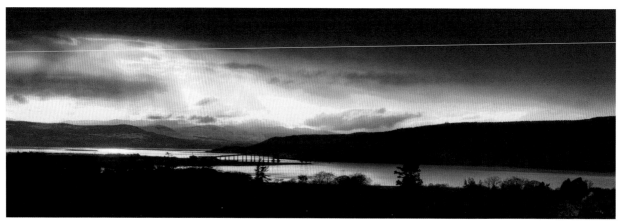

Photo by Andrew Nicholson